ff Trail

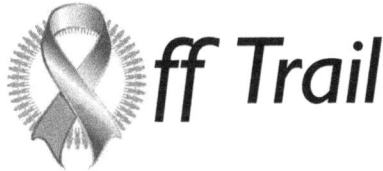

Lessons Learned from Unforeseen Breast Cancer Detours

· *Dense Tissue Concerns*
· *Rehabilitative Challenges*
· *Teenage and Family Coping*
· *Emotional and Spiritual Upheavals*
· *Possible Bilateral Mastectomy Benefits*
· *Conflicting Diagnostic Screening Recommendations*
· *Complementary Approaches to Manage Pain and Fatigue*

Jenny Glikin RN, BSN

Off Trail
Lessons Learned from Unforeseen Breast Cancer Detours

Cardinal Health Information, LLC
Copyright © 2013, by Jenny E. Glikin R.N., BSN
Inquiries can be made @ offtrailbct@gmail.com

The information in this book is the result of personal experience and research, it is not meant to replace the advice of appropriate health care providers. Every effort has been made to ensure accuracy, but listed websites or links might be altered or removed at the discretion of each organization. Referenced individuals, organizations, and institutions do not indicate endorsement or affiliation.

Cover photo by Andrew Glikin
Medical Editor: Katherine, from editavenue.com
Proofreader: Ruth Goodman, @ http://ruthgoodman.com
Book cover and interior design by Debbi Stocco, @ http://debbistocco.com

Library of Congress Catalogue Card Number: 2013905880

Includes table of contents, bibliographical references, and index.

13-ISBN: 978-0-9887095-0-8
13-ISBN: 978-0-9887095-1-5 (e-book)

Printed in the United States of America

Dedication

For you, the breast cancer survivors who are searching for answers and are in physical, emotional, spiritual, generational, parental, or marital pain—I've toiled through my own discomfort. I have met and read about some of you, but most of you I can only imagine. I hope I have served you well. Remember to follow your heart, as you too might have to explore unfamiliar trails.

And to honor your memory, Grandma, this one is also for you...

Contents

Introduction

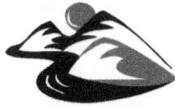

"*Do not go where the path may lead, go instead where there is no path and leave a trail.*"

— Ralph Waldo Emerson

"I have a duty to speak the truth as I see it and share not just my triumphs, not just the things that felt good, but the pain, the intense, often unmitigated pain. It is important to share how I know survival is survival and not just a walk through the rain."
— Audre Lorde

*T*hese pages do not chronicle months of chemotherapy or uncomfortable radiation treatments. My relatively early stage breast cancer diagnosis and double mastectomy kept me from needing those therapies. And yet, I still experienced temporary lymphedema, muscular dysfunctions, nerve pain, ongoing fatigue, cognitive challenges, and mobility restrictions that lasted nearly three years. It did not end there. I also developed a frozen shoulder and a capsular contracture that required additional surgery.

My combined difficulties are typically experienced by women who undergo a variety of treatments, or are at more advanced breast cancer stages, although with one important difference: I was not fighting for my life. Thanks to the luxury of time I was able to figure out what was causing the complications and I documented the evolution. Even though we undergo different treatments, our difficulties share commonalities. We might encounter similar barriers when we try to understand and manage our complications, and our bodies are bound to have a similar response to stress regardless of the stressor [111]. A small study presented at the 35th Annual San Antonio Breast Cancer Symposium (SABC) in 2012 by Dr. Bernadine Cimprich, suggests that fatigue and cognitive impairments, caused by stress *before* chemotherapy, can resemble "chemo brain" symptoms on

MRI findings, and might contribute to those deficits [76]. Aside from the physical challenges, we also have the emotional, the spiritual, and the social aspects in common.

Most of us prefer books that offer quick one-sided solutions for our health struggles. This is not one of those books. The preferred approach, though understandable and profitable, limits guidance for those of us with a medical dilemma that has different contributing factors. In other words, if you are still experiencing seemingly unrelated symptoms, long after your breast cancer treatment, and if pharmaceutical approaches have provided limited relief, read on. You won't find a magic bullet, but you will find validation, coping skills, uncommon theories, and suggestions.

Those of you with a loved one who is experiencing long-term pain and fatigue after breast cancer might also be interested. The personal account and information might help you understand that if nerve damage occurred, if a muscular imbalance has developed, if lymphedema is evident, or if long-term fatigue has become the norm your involvement is crucial. The lack of it, for a prolonged period of time, could limit your loved one's healing potential.

This is also not a tale about a breast cancer found by self-examination or from an abnormal mammogram. The cancer was unexpected and seemed atypical. A mammogram two months before my diagnosis was interpreted as normal, as it had been every other year, and I was not in a high-risk category. I lacked a strong family history, I was not overweight, I ate a low-fat diet, and I exercised frequently. I pursued an ultrasound because something felt unusual in my right breast. I was not expecting a cancer diagnosis, and most certainly not from a lesion that, according to its growth pattern, had been present for approximately 5 years. That information stunned me.

I had been under a misconception. I was certain that annual mammograms, checkups, and frequent self-examinations, would detect breast cancer at the earliest stage. Consequently part of what I am here to tell you is that those "checkups" might not be sufficient for some of us. On average, 10% to 20% of breast cancers are missed by routine mammograms, and many because of *dense tissue* [121]. Extensive dense tissue can hide cancer from a routine mammogram [14,18] and it is a *well-known risk factor* for breast cancer [30,67,176]. Some breast cancers do not calcify [14], and others feel very soft to the touch [20]. Those factors make early detection through mammograms and from manual examinations more challenging. Given those circumstances, and since my cancer developed and spread while I was premenopausal, my early *stage I* diagnosis was not the norm. Premenopausal women, who develop breast cancer and have a *lot* of breast density (BIRADS-4), are usually diagnosed at more advanced stages: IIB, III, or IV [86].

The clear connection between elevated breast density, the resulting screening difficulties, and breast cancer, has triggered a patient-driven political movement. As of July 2013 eleven states including Texas, Massachusetts, Virginia, New York and California have approved legislation to mandate information to at-risk women. Similar bills are pending in various states and at the federal level, although some medical experts fear the legislation is premature. The mandate could result in more unnecessary screenings, biopsies, and expense, rather than less, as was recommended in the fall of 2009 by the United States Preventive Services Task Force (USPSTF).

My unexpected diagnosis hurled me towards an informational roller coaster (and I've never liked roller coasters), but I felt out of control and I needed answers to make decisions. I became familiar with basic breast cancer terminology, treatment options, and reconstructive choices, although I had difficulty obtaining in-depth information on nipple-sparing mastectomies (NSM)—the 21st-century mastectomy. Many eligible women might be unaware of this seemingly rare option. The surgery offers the possibility of a better cosmetic outcome, though not all women are candidates. The option made a bilateral mastectomy less intimidating and provided a superior cosmetic outcome. The peace of mind from the aggressive surgery was an added bonus: I no longer need mammograms, MRIs, or ultrasounds, unless a recurrence episode is feared.

Even though it was helpful and necessary, most medical information felt depersonalized. My breast cancer experience did not occur during a clinical trial. It happened to me and my family, and it affected every aspect of our lives. I now know that every procedure involves an anxious woman. Every digit in the complication literature affects individuals, families, jobs, and dreams. My narrative is just one. The atypical merging of the medical saga, along with the personal impact, tries to capture the personal toll.

I wanted to help my two impressionable older teenagers through the difficult disease, treatment, and recovery terrain in store for them at such a vulnerable age. I knew the seemingly localized 1-cm lesion on my right breast would have broader emotional implications based on how we handled, or rather did not handle, my diagnosis and follow-up treatments. On different occasions I've encouraged our children to follow their hearts and listen to their instincts. I have explained that there are two sides to every story and a lesson in everything. I've reinforced that rather than simply pointing out a problem they should offer a suggestion, although above of all, I hope they will help where they see a need. Thus, the information gathered in these pages is my ultimate way of showing them I do more than just talk the talk, I also walk the walk. I hope to show other families with older teens that it is possible to thrive through a breast cancer diagnosis, not just cope.

Yes, I set out to do breast cancer *right* for our children, a lofty goal that wound up having an alternate agenda. I verified that our children have always been and will always be my greatest teachers. If I am not sure how to proceed in a difficult situation, the answer is clear when I approach it from the perspective of their learning potential. I was determined to show them how to handle hardship, how to continue to enjoy life under stress, and how to be open to the gifts that can be found in adversity. Instead, and quite unexpectedly, they became my unlikely tutors and I their grateful apprentice.

By now, you must have noticed that I consider the emotions from a cancer experience, to be as critical as the physical toll. Well before the scalpel makes its appearance, and long after it has left its mark, the emotional environment sets the tone for individuals, families, and friends. Every person participates, but it's those of us with cancer who must captain our emotional ships through rough waters, towards positive realistic shores. If you've already experienced cancer you know that our loved ones prefer we return to our pre-cancer *normal* as soon as possible. That is understandable, but if we continue to experience difficulties their expectations become unrealistic, and our different needs can cause friction. Try to keep in mind that with calm, honest, and mutual communication, we can help strengthen our relationships, rather than letting cancer weaken them.

Since my stepson's favorite mantra set me on the right path, I want to share it with you. Andrew has long believed our attitude is the *one* variable we can control in any situation, particularly a difficult one. That concept guided me many times. The tone between my needs and those of my loved ones had to be genuine, otherwise they would see through me; they know me so well. The balance was difficult. I did not always accomplish it, but I kept trying. For better or for worse, my breast cancer experience was a learning-teaching opportunity.

I naively anticipated a linear recovery. I tried to work with three physical therapists, a pain specialist, and with a program for cancer survivors, although nerve disruptions excluded me. For these reasons, this endeavor is also not a tale about how traditional mobility recommendations were instrumental. A year and a half after my initial surgery I was getting worse, not better. Effective suggestions to help rehabilitate my left arm, shoulder, back, and neck to some semblance of normality were sparser once weakness and muscular imbalances developed from the nerve damage. Mine was not an uncommon experience. "Rehabilitation problems are common after breast cancer surgeries." [31]

As I began the lengthy task of understanding my difficulties, information on a broader scale began to emerge. Many other women experience some type of long-term pain after breast cancer treatment [142]. Yes, I said women. As a rule, those studies do not include men with the disease [78]. The umbrella term to describe those unwelcome events, which can result from every type of surgery and follow-up therapy, is *post breast therapy pain syndrome* (PBTPS) [142].

Don't despair. Progress has been made, thanks to innovative techniques. Modified mastectomies that spare important muscles have lowered the frequency. Procedures that preserve key nerves [78], and specific nerve blocks before surgery, seem to lessen the likelihood of long-term pain [82]. Surgery related pain is lower with *sentinel lymph node biopsies* (the removal of just a few lymph nodes), compared to *axillary lymph node dissections* (many lymph nodes removed on the affected side), which were the norm a few years ago [100]. Assuming the right therapies are combined, even women with limited lymph node involvement might be able to safely keep most of their lymph nodes [62,117].

The progress should reassure the newly diagnosed but also encourage self-involvement. Even though surgical complications have been lessened, and less invasive techniques are becoming the norm, 47% to 50% of us continue to experience some degree of pain months or years after our treatment ends [59,103]. Aside from pain caused by chemical therapies, or due to nerve damage from surgery, muscular imbalances and scar tissue might be keeping some survivors in pain. We have to become proactive. Since some of those pain scenarios can be prevented or unraveled, our active involvement might lower yet another high breast cancer survivor statistic: 10% to 30% of women who undergo surgery for breast cancer develop chronic pain [142,133].

It is not clear which surgical treatment is responsible for the majority of long-term pain in breast cancer patients. While many have long believed that mastectomies are the biggest culprit [142], more recent data shows that young age, radiation therapy, and having a lot of lymph nodes removed seem to have more of an impact than the choice of surgery, particularly if they are combined [59,82].

In all fairness, conducting research on pain after breast cancer must be challenging. Every therapy is capable of causing pain. Pain is hard to measure, and without a nationalized health care data base, gathering data in the United States must be difficult. Our healing potential varies, and since women living alone are more prone to these pain syndromes, some experts believe psychological aspects are contributing. I believe there might be another explanation. Those women have less assistance and might need to overstrain, which I know increases pain.

If we continue to experience pain, or if we face rehabilitative challenges, the multiple built-in barriers can seem daunting. Nerve pain defies medical understanding, and prescription pharmaceuticals continue to be the chosen treatment [126]. Regrettably, they cannot reverse nerve damage, they have multiple side effects, and many of us find their benefit limited. Muscle relaxants are a Band-Aid solution for muscular imbalances, but they too have undesirable effects without addressing the root of the problem. Aside from those factors, and to add insult to injury, I was unable to tolerate several pharmaceuticals.

Out of desperation I ventured away from my preconceived medical trail, into complementary medicine. Those approaches lowered my pain, but seemingly unrelated imbalances were keeping my muscles painfully weak, affecting my concentration, and prolonging my fatigue. Those challenges responded to a combination of traditional medicine and complementary approaches. Prior to this experience I would have considered the tactics I used unorthodox. Not anymore. On more than one occasion I arrived at the juncture where desperation meets experimentation. Those of you who are or have been there might relate. When quality of life is compromised, atypical considerations are investigated. Pain and fatigue syndromes are difficult to manage and even more challenging to experience. Hence, I feel a sense of responsibility to share what worked for me.

I am not a doctor, or a physical therapist, or a massage therapist, or a complementary health care provider, but we did work together. To understand what was happening to my body, I picked all of their brains for their expertise; without them I would not have been able to do much on my own. I do not claim to have the answers to all of these complicated riddles. What worked for me may not work for somebody else. As you read keep in mind that the information I present is not meant to replace medical dialogue, it is intended to enhance those discussions.

Not all of my experiences were negative. This story has uplifting angles. In many respects, these have been some of the best years of my life. I like the person who emerged better than the one I was before breast cancer. My relationships were tested but ultimately strengthened. My priorities were shifted in a positive manner, and I became a breast cancer advocate. When pain and weakness made it impossible to work and I could no longer perform routine tasks, I turned my forced isolation into an opportunity for research, introspection, and writing. I was transformed physically, emotionally, psychologically, and most surprisingly, spiritually.

The latter occurred because spiritual guidance played a role from the onset. The occurrences were very different, but they felt more real than previous experiences. I realized that even though I could not understand them, and since I wanted to benefit, it was best to accept the insights unconditionally. My spiritual perspective inevitably changed—for the first time I learned to accept abstract concepts. Initially, I looked for spiritual strength to help my family cope and to shelter them from pain, but once again, I benefitted the most. I kept those experiences in these pages. Without them, my breast cancer picture would lack its most brilliant colors.

Learning to listen to my intuition was one of the many gifts of forced introspection. Therefore, I want to remind all of you to listen to your intuition. It is there, just pay attention. After a while I learned to tell the difference between fear and intuition. Intuition is not panic; it is subtle, it is constant, and it is wise. My intuition would more easily manifest itself during meditation and time alone. When I was faced with difficult choices, I researched information, spoke with the experts, and then I paid attention to my instincts. My educated instinctual decisions were proven right on more than one occasion—beyond coincidence. One of those instances was my surgical choice. Initially a double mastectomy seemed too aggressive but in time it proved appropriate. Intuition made me pursue seemingly unnecessary screenings, and by extension, a timely diagnosis. Like I said, my experience was atypical from the start.

A few disclaimers are well overdue. Even though I worked as a registered nurse for ten years, I do not have a current professional résumé. Thanks to this project I understand my second language better than I did before breast cancer, but English composition was not part of my formal education; thus, I have struggled with that aspect. I'm also not a writer by trade; in fact, I am a lousy typist. When I started documenting my thoughts, it was not with the intent of writing a book. Had I not become concerned about how similar difficulties affect other survivors, I wouldn't have aspired to that goal. My only claim is that I am a breast cancer survivor who experienced and conquered many hurdles.

My unexpected challenges led to the type of self-involvement that we all need in a complex health crisis. I asked informed questions, I listened to my body, and

I became an active participant in my care. I set out to understand *why* I was not well. Since I often felt like I was on undocumented territory, I researched barriers, personalized an approach, and I recorded my successes and my failures. My perseverance paid off in every way, thanks to my relentless quest for answers, and because I refused to believe my difficulties were permanent.

Consequently I want to encourage all of you to become familiar with *self-advocacy*. Even if you are not a health care professional you can still advocate for yourself. Only you can listen to the cues your body provides each and every day. We can enhance our health care dialogue and care by identifying and understanding our symptoms before going to our appointments. That type of patient involvement has been labeled *participatory medicine* [115]. Medical partnerships are particularly welcome in *integrative* medical settings, where traditional and complementary medical knowledge is combined.

The various hurdles created frustration, but lawsuits are out of the question. Remember, much is unknown in the field of breast cancer. I was not exempt from complications, I simply experienced several difficulties. Besides, every delay had a hidden purpose that might not have been fulfilled without the added time factors. All of the health care providers who crossed my path are healers in more ways than they know. Each provided a key piece towards the completion of my complex puzzle. Even those who refused to believe me or felt I would not get better helped. They forced me to become more involved.

Instead of lawsuits, we need to find a way to reinstate medical dialogue. *Interactive discussions have been lost in the quest for patient privacy and with specialized medicine.* Limited or no access to patients' medical records, due to electronic incompatibilities, makes it nearly impossible to piece together complex scenarios with specialty overlaps, as happened in the management of my complications. At one point 7 medical offices had part of my medical information, but none had it all. When phone interviews were conducted by a National Cancer Institute center, on cancer patients who felt "something went wrong" in their care, nearly half felt communication "breakdowns" had been part of their experience [96]. Dialogue between traditional health care providers, complementary medicine professionals, and their integrative medical counterparts, also needs to be enhanced. When we've exhausted our medical options, and our quality of life is still poor, 80% of cancer patients resort to some type of complementary health care modality [60].

Frequent lawsuits distract from the problems in our health care system. Aside from creating more communication barriers, additional expense, and unnecessary testing, they confine practitioners to therapies that can be defended in court; unfortunately, some of us do not respond to those approaches. Several physician friends and my 23-year marriage to a doctor have made me aware of these issues. Sadly we've lost some of those friends to the high physician suicide rate in the United States. Doctorswithdepression.org claims "the trend is alarming." The multiple unknowns, the built-in barriers, and the constant legal threats, make the unrealistic standard of perfection most of us expect impossible. All of us will need good healthcare and good dialogue between those practitioners someday, but if technical, financial, and legal barriers remain the norm, frustrated capable physician will continue to abandon the profession. Anticipated physician shortages will worsen. Our health—or the health of a loved one—could suffer.

Insufficient medical dialogue could explain why post breast therapy pain syndrome "is not well recognized by physicians." [142] The practitioners who are aware might lack clear guidelines or the ability to make effective referrals: in 2007, there were less than 50 physicians in the United States with cancer rehabilitation training [31]. That leaves primary physicians, but most are not versed in the management of cancer complications. It is easy to assume that our troubles are either mild or psychosomatic. That is not the case. The much-preferred image of the happy-go-lucky survivor needs defying. It is inaccurate for some of us, even if we've been granted a reprieve from our diagnosis, try to stay positive, and derive a lot of meaning from our experience.

Aside from pain complications, other issues need attention. In *After the Cure: The Untold Stories of Breast Cancer Survivors*, Drs. Abel and Subramanian conducted a study to get a sense of lingering, long-term side effects. They found that chronic fatigue and cognitive impairments, from chemotherapy and radiation, were the most frequent and disruptive symptoms. A few survivors found complementary therapies beneficial but unaffordable without insurance recognition, while others were hesitant because they were not endorsed by health care providers. Since complications were not always acknowledged by medical teams, some women could not receive disability benefits. Others had less disabling symptoms but were still forced to change careers. To better manage or reduce complications, the foreword contributor Dr. Patricia Ganz, M.D., advocates for more research, even though the various symptoms would be difficult to measure [3]. Disabilities might be higher in low-income patients; their unemployment rate could be as high as 30% five years after treatment [175].

The need to cope with residual complications is welcome; it is the result of medical advances. Since the phenomenon is relatively new these days there are more breast cancer survivors in the United States, maybe as many as 2.5 million [3]. On the flip side a management gap has been created—complication research has not progressed at the same pace as treatment [78].

Further research on pain caused by breast cancer treatment has been suggested [142,153]. Additional investigations could help determine why so many complications develop, may improve rehabilitation outcomes, and could result in more effective pain relief interventions. Healthcare practitioner awareness and patient education would inevitably result. Large cancer centers and organizations hold informative meetings and have comprehensive websites, but many of us need individualized assistance for a prolonged period of time.

Change might be on the horizon. Thanks to various complementary health care providers, and because of progressive integrative oncologists, a specialty is starting to emerge for lingering survivorship issues. Specific complementary approaches, such as acupuncture and mind-body techniques have proven helpful [24,107], although perhaps because they are not widely recognized, most insurance companies do not provide those benefits. The growing number of reputable cancer centers that are offering integrative care, along with more complication awareness, should enhance quality of life for many survivors, from different types of cancers.

Traditional medical experts are also addressing these complex issues. The first that comes to mind is Dr. Andrea Cheville, M.D. Thanks to an informative article she co-authored [31], I began to understand some of my rehabilitative barriers. The second is Dr. Marissa Weiss M.D., a champion of survivorship issues. She is the founder of two important organizations: breastcancer.org and lbbc.org (Living Beyond Breast Cancer). Dr. Weiss is also the co-author of *Living Well Beyond Breast Cancer,* where she acknowledges that many difficulties can linger. She provides useful self-involvement suggestions, including how to choose health care providers, as well as detailed information on pharmaceuticals to manage long-term pain [171]. I have not met those experts, but I am indebted to them. They reinforced that through reading, we can sometimes bridge life's trying junctures.

We can do our part. Aside from developing a better understanding of our medical conditions, we can facilitate medical record transfers. If at all possible, you should obtain your cancer treatment and follow-up care at a major cancer center. They are more likely to share information electronically, many of them offer integrative programs, and a lot of them have specialized support staff, should complications arise.

I hope to contribute by sharing my research with those of you who lack the time, the ability to interpret medical literature, or the resources I was fortunate to have. Since they so frequently overlap with quality of life topics (and detailed data can be difficult to access), I also share information on recurrence statistics, self-advocacy issues, and treatment choices, among other things. I present practical suggestions and information throughout the account, but most of the research is in the advocacy segment, the last portion.

Just like many others familiar with the medical field, I used to enjoy piecing together a medical riddle. But let me tell you, I've now seen the flip side of that coin. None applies when the challenge involves a diagnosis, a report, or a statistic with the potential to cut your own life short—the experience is more than clinical. The multiple levels of the experience could explain why my husband found it difficult to cope with the medical aspects of my diagnosis, and why my journal entries range between attempts at putting my medical puzzle together, emotional outbursts on both sides of the spectrum, and spiritual bewilderment.

If you encounter a difficult health detour, you too might want to consider journaling and researching. The efforts provided an outlet, empowered me, and kept me focused and organized. My journal felt like a friend; I missed it when I did not make an entry for several days. The blog and journal provide glimpses into the often difficult aftermath of a cancer diagnosis. Both sections show my decisions for what they were—a series of personal choices. The combination of cancer stage, health, age, financial resources, support systems, personal beliefs, and work circumstances should personalize decisions. The time sequence gives a sense of how we as a family handled the challenges, our emotions, our attempted coping skills, and it illustrates how my complications and conclusions evolved.

Sometimes progress is slower than expected, but we might feel less isolated if we know that others are going through a similar ordeal. One breast cancer survivor made me feel less alone when she shared that her experience was "the loneliest journey" she has ever traveled. She was experiencing pain and mobility challenges, but she too found it difficult to find solutions. With the intent of offering validation and information to those of you with similar mobility riddles, I've tried to share what worked for me, along with information on each topic. My contribution to the cause is bound to be limited—many issues need attention and each is very complex. Even so, a sense of responsibility to help in some manner remains and refuses to be ignored.

I will conclude this introductory portion with a clarification. The wish to help other survivors is not uniquely mine, not by any stretch of the imagination. It is the golden thread binding all breast cancer survivors together. It symbolizes our constant readiness to help each other regardless of age, economics, or cultural background. That sense of interconnectedness is one of the most positive aspects of this difficult experience.

Part One

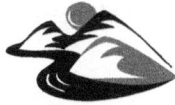

<u>Intuition</u>

The ability to acquire knowledge without inference or the use of reason. The word "intuition" comes from the Latin word intueri, which is often translated as having the meaning of "to look inside" or to "contemplate."

(Wikipedia)

DIAGNOSIS, DECISIONS, AND SURGERY PREPARATIONS

"The only real valuable thing is intuition."
— Albert Einstein

"Trusting our intuition often saves us from disaster."
— Anne Wilson Schaef

That morning, when I woke up with my left hand protectively cupped over my right breast, was in the midst of an unusually cool December. At that instant between sleep and wakefulness I experienced a seemingly trivial sensation. The feeling was vague and it could have been ignored, except this was the third time I experienced it over a six-week period. The slight itch lasted just a few seconds, though it was still familiar. It reminded me of when I needed to express more breast milk for the sake of comfort, even though my babies had finished their nursing session.

I did not understand why I was experiencing those nearly forgotten sensations. They only made sense when I was told that my breast cancer originated and spread, through the inner spaces of my milk ducts. How could I have known that those sensations, which I had not experienced for 14 years, would play a key role in obtaining a timely diagnosis? No, I did not have a palpable mass, discharge, or redness. I was not experiencing pain, although my dense tissue felt a little different. I showed my husband Sandy the area in question, and he arrived at a very logical conclusion: I should not be concerned.

◈

A NORMAL MAMMOGRAM & ADDITIONAL SCREENINGS

I still scheduled a mammogram, even though it was such a busy time. Sandy had been unexpectedly hospitalized for 10 days, it had just been our son's birthday, our kids were home from school, and Sandy was still recuperating. And yet, when the scheduler asked if I could go in the next day, I jumped at the chance.

I was not concerned. Three pregnancies, the first of which was at the age of 29, and nursing my babies for two years had lowered my risk. My annual checkup the month before had been normal, just like every year, and only one second-degree relative had been diagnosed with breast cancer. I did not smoke, or drink in excess, I did frequent breast exams, and my Hispanic ethnicity also lessened the odds. Even so, I had a mammogram on December 23rd—a day I usually don't venture out. The technician did not see anything out of the ordinary, even though additional films were taken. She stressed that I should not be alarmed, but if I needed more reassurance an *ultrasound* or a *diagnostic* mammogram would be more in depth. The report was not delayed because of the holidays, not at all. As usual, the results were in my mailbox the following week. The report not only read *normal,* it explained there was no *evidence of cancer.*

The moment when I considered filing the report but didn't is still vivid. Why didn't I? For the first time I wanted more testing. A similar ambivalence had crossed my mind two years prior, with a *dense tissue throughout the right breast* report. I made very limited inquiries. The partial data led me to assume that, for women under the age of 50, dense tissue is normal, thickened breast tissue. Had I explored the subject in depth, I would have learned that dense is not only considered a *strong* risk factor for breast cancer [30,86,104], but that my high percentage could make an early-stage diagnosis with mammograms more difficult [20].

An earlier-stage diagnosis, without infiltration, would have given me a better long-term prognosis. If fewer lymph nodes had been biopsied, the likelihood of my eventual nerve damage would have also been lessened. This time I did not leave well enough alone. I pursued an ultrasound, even though I had no rational explanation for doing so, other than perhaps peace of mind.

Getting approval for an ultrasound was not difficult—my physician had already experienced cancer. I later thanked him for letting me follow my instincts; I know women who have been denied additional screenings. I understand the resistance. Before my unlikely diagnosis I shared the same concerns. Since I had no symptoms, I could have been told that the screening was not necessary, I was not in a high-risk category, it might cause unnecessary worrying, further testing can lead to a negative biopsy, and additional screenings increase health care costs.

Health care professionals need guidelines, but where does my roundabout way of getting diagnosed fit into that equation? I don't know. But my perspective now includes less-conventional thinking; our bodies are capable of sending signals we often dismiss, and disregarding them can be a mistake. I know there are no clinical trials to back up such a theory, and that scientific guidelines must derive from clinical studies. But I also know that if medical guidelines had been my only consideration on that day when my mammogram report should have been filed away and was not, things would have turned out quite differently for me.

Ultrasounds are not invasive procedures. The technician simply moved a gelled probe over my right breast, while I relaxed on a stretcher. I apologized as I pointed out the area in question—I could not locate the slightly irregular area I had been able to palpate just the previous week. From either wishful thinking or from force of habit, I anticipated going home afterwards. I was sure the usual "normal" report would arrive in the mail, but that would not happen. Instead, a *diagnostic* mammogram was ordered. This screening involves a lot more pressure and views, though perhaps for those reasons it was able to penetrate through my dense tissue.

That was not the last concerning experience. Once the technician referred to the area as a lump, I was guided towards a film collection. The radiologist pointed to one mass visible on ultrasound images, but not on mammogram views—those only showed my dense tissue. She explained that the edges of one mass were suspicious, based on the color a cyst could be ruled out, and that the area had not *pressed* out as it should have on the diagnostic mammogram. A biopsy was recommended.

At last I had Sandy's attention. He tried to reassure me by reminding me that 80% of breast biopsies are negative [28]. We agreed to keep to ourselves what had been recommended, at least until the biopsy report became available. It seemed necessary to discuss how we would handle a breast cancer diagnosis, including that it would be best to keep it from our mothers for as long as possible. We were not aware of it then, and perhaps it was better that way, but our breast cancer roller coaster had officially begun.

I didn't research. I thought I was an unlikely candidate. Ignorance can feel like bliss; the possibility of a positive outcome remains when all is not known, although instead of ecstasy, the period was the calm before my oncoming storm.

There was one exception. Five days before the biopsy I felt an overwhelming need to leave town. I blamed the impulse on the stressful events of the previous month. In addition to Sandy's hospitalization, along with three invasive procedures for unexpected bleeding, my mother was recuperating from a week long hospitalization, and only two weeks before, a dear friend committed suicide. These words clearly came to mind: "I'd better get out of town while I still can." Within a matter of minutes I made reservations, and Sandy and I left the very next day. The getaway was timely. It strengthened us for the oncoming train that was just around the corner, and a year and a half would elapse before I would experience a semblance of traveling comfort.

࿇

BIOPSY & UNEXPLAINABLE EXPERIENCES

There is a blissful mental place where repetitive motion meets controlled breathing. It is a type of meditative relaxation that can result from various exercises, including yoga. The morning before the biopsy I chose to run to ease my anxiety, although on that morning the outcome was very different, quite unusual, and rather overwhelming.

Since the experience was a sensation it is very hard to put into words, but words are all I have; I will have to give them a try. As I was in that familiar sense of relaxation, I began to feel enveloped by a fatherly being, conveying unconditional love. I am certain of that specific sensation, even though I have very few memories of paternal love. The perception was clear and overpowering. I had never experienced anything so vivid, although it was as brief as it was overwhelming. When Sandy saw me on my knees in tears, he assumed I was sensing the stress of the upcoming biopsy. I tried to explain, but he could not understand. How could he? I could barely understand it myself. I should have understood. My biopsy would reveal cancer, although at the time I was too overwhelmed to make the obvious connection.

The biopsy was ultrasound-guided and not uncomfortable. What was uncomfortable was the *hematoma* I developed. In other words, a pocket of blood formed under my skin. Although the discomfort could not be blamed on the bleeding, it was from the pressure applied to my chest to stop it. The hematoma was significant. It was still visible a month later when I went to surgery, and the bruising was still noticeable weeks after my double mastectomy. The procedure was performed on a Thursday morning, but we would not learn the result until the following Tuesday. The period was surreal. Internally my life was essentially on hold, while externally I was trying to pretend that nothing had changed.

I did not have to wait five days. On the following Sunday I knew I had cancer the instant I opened my eyes. The cancer certainty felt very out of place. I had slept well, and my dreams did not indicate cancer concerns. I'm glad I was alone. My family would have wondered why I seemed to be carrying out an angry, desperate discussion on my own. The dialogue is nearly impossible to describe; although one side of the conversation was internal, I was not generating it. Even so, the message was explicit, scary, and reassuring all at once; I definitely had cancer, I would eventually be well and cancer-free, it was a gift not a punishment, and the gift would have many layers.

My perception of loneliness was beyond physical. I was already sensing that cancer would be a personal experience, even though others would be there to help and sympathize. My tears continued for what felt like an eternity, except in reality only two hours elapsed. I felt like a child begging to be spared. After a while I realized what every child in that position must eventually realize—crying does not change the inevitable. Yes, I was glad for the solitude. Crying had been necessary, but it would have been concerning to others. In their presence I would have restrained my tears.

The road before me seemed daunting, but spiritual support promised to ease the way. The dialogue, along with the experience before the biopsy, provided encouragement for years, although words cannot explain to what extent. They were humbling, reassuring, and they kept me in a state of awe. I knew they had occurred—I just did not believe I deserved to be their recipient. Without the promise of a full recovery I would have stopped looking for answers prematurely.

⚜

RELAYING THE NEWS

I first shared the news with our youngest children, Neil and Nicole. The order might seem odd, but I was hoping to show them that spiritual guidance exists. Besides, without a medical report Sandy would have approached the situation with humor, and my intended message would have been lost. They were not sure what to make of it all. They only understood it 48 hours later with the official report. Since she was sent to speak with a counselor, Nicole must have been upset at school. Neil, true to his nature, was far more composed, although that also concerned me. I asked his close friends to help him vent his feelings. They are both lucky. Their friends provided comfort when I could not.

Extended family members were next. My youngest brother, Hernan, was a good place to start. Only he knew about the biopsy and I needed his spiritual comfort; besides, I did not want to have a discussion with a spiritual skeptic who would doubt my certainty. Alfredo, my oldest brother, was next in line for similar reasons, but the stress of worrying them was oppressive. It took me two days to gather the courage to call my other siblings, Carlos and Diana, and four weeks elapsed before we spoke with our mothers, although we wanted to reassure them with a treatment plan. Sharing the news with my mother was difficult. The pain in her eyes was clear. From her perspective the negative news were flowing in the wrong direction.

There was still one more person I had to confront on that sad Sunday—my husband when he came home from work. In the evening I gave Sandy a calm rendition of what I had already told our teens, even though I knew it sounded crazy. Clearly, I was unable to grasp the meaning of what I was saying, but each promise fulfilled itself in its own way, and in its own time.

I was at a meeting and missed the anticipated call. Sandy wanted me to call the answering service, even though he does not like to disturb doctors at home. I did not make the call. I knew it would not bring reassurances. The next morning my doctor insisted we meet to discuss the results. I declined. I already knew what the report would reveal, I was calm and not alone, and I wanted to start making the unavoidable appointments. He explained the diagnosis could have been far worse: the cancer was *well differentiated*, a slow growing, *low-grade* tumor.

A medical team that gives you a sense of personal connection is worth seeking. I did not want to feel like a medical record number. Shortly after the unwelcome call our phone rang yet again. It was a friend from our Sunday school carpool who, unbeknownst to me, worked with the recommended surgeon. That thoughtful friend arranged my initial oncology appointment within 48 hours, answered many panicked questions, suggested a plastic surgeon, and made a couple of house calls after surgery. Medical care does not get any more personal than that.

⁂

DECISIONS: LUMPECTOMY VS. A SINGLE MASTECTOMY VS. DOUBLE MASTECTOMY. RECONSTRUCTIVE CHOICES & NIPPLE-SPARING MASTECTOMY

There were so many decisions that needed to be made, that sometimes I felt I could drown from the stress of it all. Numbers and statistics frequently marched across my computer screen. One of them was the slightly less than 5% recurrence rate over a five-year period for my stage I of the disease [104]. In personal terms that translated into having a 95% chance of watching my children graduate from high school. It also meant that 5 out of 100 of us will never see that 5-year mark. Other statistics were less encouraging. According to the American Cancer Society, a little over 250,000 new breast cancer diagnoses and close to 40,000 deaths from the disease were predicted in the United States for the 2009 calendar year. I tried to cope with the information overload by making lists, by setting priorities, and by creating a folder with information and personal notes.

Several breast cancer survivors emphasized that life would eventually resume a normal rhythm. A friend, who is also a professional in the cancer field, shared an important fact: in medical literature a recurrence is only labeled that way if the cancer is on the *same breast,* but not on the *opposite breast*, and in some instances, a cancer episode on the same breast is not considered a recurrence [171]. That information made me look at the recurrence statistics with some degree of hesitation. I would consider a new cancer lesion an unwelcome event, regardless of the type or the location.

I also learned that insurance companies have a legal mandate to pay for reconstructions and surgeries to achieve symmetry after mastectomies. The federal mandate includes procedures on the opposite breast, treatment for complications such as lymphedema, as well as prosthetic inserts. Co-pays and deductibles need to be met, plan restrictions apply, and state-to-state insurance laws can vary [28].

Even though it is a daunting task, you too will need to understand your cancer data to make informed surgical decisions. I will only mention the basic "prognostic indicators" because they are so important, but such information needs to come from your oncologists and is well explained in patient resources. Besides, there are others and new ones are emerging. A good place to start is to know the size of your tumor, the *estrogen and progesterone receptor status* (if female hormones encourage cancer growth), if it infiltrated, and if the cancer is *HER2-positive*, which might indicate a more aggressive cancer. Factors such as a strong family history and young age at diagnosis might prompt *BRCA1* or *BRCA2* genetic testing, although you and your oncologist will discuss all of that in detail.

Breast-conservation surgery (or lumpectomy) would have been a poor choice due to unpredictable surgical findings, but initially it was considered a good option. Had I been a candidate, the surgery would have been followed by radiation and aromatase inhibitors (postmenopausal anti-estrogen therapy) for several years, because my cancer was estrogen-receptor positive (ER+). Through personal inquiries, we confirmed that breast-conservation surgery is typically recommended for what appeared to be an isolated, infiltrated mass. Meanwhile, I knew that after breast-conservation surgery many women, particularly small-breasted women, seek plastic surgery, including implants, to recreate their lost symmetry. And to regain their own sense of symmetry, large-breasted women sometimes have the noncancerous breast reduced. Some patients go back to surgery within days or weeks to achieve *cancer-free margins*, and some wind up with a mastectomy after all. I did not want to be in that position. As it turns out, I would have been.

The combination of breast-conservation surgery, implants, and a lot of dense tissue seemed like a bad idea. I was afraid implants would limit mammogram compression on my already difficult to interpret dense tissue. Besides, breast density can make screenings after breast cancer more challenging [74]. Even my recent menopause had to be considered. Those of us who still have a lot of dense tissue after menopause have an increased risk of breast cancer [86].

Once I ruled out breast-conservation surgery, the next choice was between a *unilateral and a bilateral mastectomy*. At that point I had to consider that my lesion, based on its size and growth pattern, had been repeatedly missed, even though it should have been noticed years prior on a routine mammogram. In other words, if I chose a one-sided mastectomy, a recurrence might be difficult to detect by mammogram or by self-exams on the opposite breast.

There were also cosmetic issues to consider, even though it all seemed overwhelming, but depending on my initial choice that outcome could vary. When both plastic surgeons explained how difficult it is to match an artificial breast to a natural one, I started leaning towards a double mastectomy. A bilateral reconstruction without radiation could also provide enhanced symmetry. The radiation I would receive if I chose the lumpectomy, and later needed a mastectomy, would make my skin and muscles less pliable. Radiation can also increase the incidence of developing a *capsular contracture* (a lot of scar tissue around an implant), a complication that often requires surgery. As a nurse I had taken care of several patients with radiation-related injuries and that too scared me, even though the likelihood is less frequent.

I began to lose my allegiance towards my breast tissue. Keeping even part of it suddenly felt like a liability. It would keep me nervous about future screenings and could interfere with the best possible cosmetic outcome. The bilateral mastectomy decision was less intimidating when I realized that my breast tissue was no longer necessary. It had already fulfilled its nursing purpose 14 years prior.

From a reconstructive perspective, an *implant reconstruction* seemed like my best option. A *tissue-transplant reconstruction* was ruled out because of my low weight, but those surgeries are a good choice if the area in question has received radiation, if a lot of skin is lost from a mastectomy, or for women who wish to avoid implants and the need to replace them at a later date. Since muscles and skin are typically transferred, from either the back or from the abdominal areas, tissue-transplant reconstructions require a longer recovery time. My inability to contemplate too many reconstructive options was welcome—I was already on information overload.

A key factor in the double mastectomy decision was my eligibility for a *nipple-sparing mastectomy* (NSM). The option was offered by my internationally renowned breast surgeon and my experienced plastic surgeon. I was a good candidate. I was small breasted and my cancer was located away from the nipple area. That surgery would leave my entire skin surface and my nipples intact, and the incisions would be at my natural breast crease instead of across my chest. I've since learned that eligibility for this procedure varies. I might not have been a candidate at another facility, although my breast surgeon did explain that a different procedure would be performed if my surgical findings deemed it necessary.

The NSM procedure was pioneered at the Cleveland Clinic by Dr. Joseph P. Crowe, M.D. It is typically performed on women with a *genetic* predisposition as a preventive measure. The use of the technique on early-stage, *nonhereditary* breast cancer is relatively new. Long-term research is limited, although studies over 10 years seem promising from a safety perspective [39,160]. Saving just the skin with a *skin-sparing* mastectomy (SSM) is considered safer than procedures that preserve the nipple. Overall, traditional mastectomies that remove the nipple and a lot of skin remain the gold standard, for those of us who choose or need a mastectomy [125].

There are surgical risks. Sometimes the nipple necroses. In simpler terms it loses its blood supply, does not adhere, and needs to be removed. Lost nipple sensation is the norm, but new techniques to save important nerves might change that outcome for some women, although lack of sensation might happen with any type of mastectomy. Many breast surgeons consider the procedure risky—they neither suggest it nor perform it. NSM "leaves potentially harmful cells behind." [151] In 2009, only 25 surgeons in the United States were performing the procedure. Only 5% of mastectomies were the nipple-sparing kind, even though 20% to 30% of women who had a mastectomy were eligible [108].

As I said, criteria varies from institution to institution, but generally, women who are not at an early enough stage, are very large breasted, have large tumors, have cancers in proximity to the nipple or near the skin are not eligible. Other factors might also play a role. More and more hospitals are offering NSM as an option and the research is growing. If this procedure is chosen, finding an experienced surgeon is extremely important.

I was still not done. I had to choose either the *one-step* reconstructive procedure with an *immediate reconstruction,* or the lengthier process with expanders that would take several weeks. With the one-step process, the implants would be inserted under the upper layer of my pectoral muscles immediately after the mastectomy, and with no further surgeries. That seemed attractive at first, until both plastic surgeons emphasized the cosmetic outcome could be inferior.

Through all of the stress I started to suspect my strength of character and my determination surpassed my preconceived boundaries. Yes, my appearance was important enough to pursue the lengthier reconstructive process, but the outcome would *not* define me. It is possible those sentiments would have been different if I doubted Sandy's loyalty or if I had been younger. Other survivors, in a similar circumstance, recognized that even though we were given a breast cancer diagnosis, we were still fortunate. Our cosmetic outcome did not have the power to take away what mattered in our lives.

Wait, I should backtrack just a little. I want to elaborate on one of my surgical choices. Aside from increasing complication awareness, I've tried to gather information on out-of-the-norm breast cancer topics. One of those is on a surgery that is growing in popularity—even among those of us without a genetic predisposition—the choice of a double mastectomy.

※

WHY ARE SO MANY OF US CHOOSING TO HAVE OUR HEALTHY BREAST REMOVED? (CONTRALATERAL PROPHYLACTIC MASTECTOMY OR CPM) WHAT ARE THE POSSIBLE BENEFITS?

No one should tell you what to do if you have the luxury to choose your breast cancer treatment. Yes, I am a little biased, but I've been there and done that. I've tried to decipher the overall survival (OS), the recurrence, and the quality of life statistics. I have spoken with others in a similar circumstance, and I've read about how different physicians feel about the most difficult choice: how aggressive to be after a breast cancer diagnosis.

Taking advantage of the referenced material might help you understand this surgical choice, assuming you want to explore the possible benefits. If you are interested, the gathered data could save you valuable time. Detailed information on this option can be difficult to access. Besides, stress confuses research and makes the data we are given hard to understand and remember.

CPM surgery rates have increased by 150% since 1998 [90], a trend that is concerning to some specialists. While a few studies have shown a slight survival benefit over a 10 to 20-year period [70,118,163], most studies show that double mastectomies do not improve survival rates [35,54,122]. Even so, many women without a genetic predisposition, which account for only 5% to 10% of breast cancers, and those at the earliest breast cancer stages, are choosing the surgery [90]. Patient preferences are playing a role, but many experts are still against the concept of removing a healthy breast without a genetic risk. It has been theorized that we are making our choice based on our overestimation of the benefit [54,64], yet another reason to address this seemingly taboo topic.

A basic understanding of recurrence terminology might be a good place to start. There are *same* or *ipsilateral* breast tumor recurrences (IBTR), and then there is cancer on the *opposite* or *contralateral* breast (CBC), although cancer on the opposite breast is considered a new cancer, not necessarily a recurrence. A new cancer (or a *second primary*) can also happen on the already treated breast, and it too might be excluded from recurrence statistics [171]. Another unwelcome event is a *regional* recurrence, which might be noticed under the arm or above the clavicle and can involve nearby muscles or bones. Then there is the most dreaded recurrence of all—*metastatic* breast cancer. The different terminology makes it hard to understand the term *recurrence*. Try to keep detailed records. If a recurrence occurs, even decades later, the documentation can help differentiate a new cancer from a true recurrence.

For the sake of simplicity, and because both might be lessened by CPM, I will only address *local* recurrences and *contralateral* (opposite breast) cancers. A local recurrence can be a new or a second cancer, and it surfaces on remaining breast tissue, skin, or close to a mastectomy site without further spread. I will mention each side separately. Remember, figures are influenced by personal cancer data, and most of these episodes are effectively treated without compromising longevity. Longevity can be reduced when a second lumpectomy is chosen, rather than a mastectomy on the already treated side [162], and with repeated recurrences [6].

To determine possible local recurrences (on the affected side), statistics between breast-conservation surgeries and *single*-sided mastectomies should be considered, although that is difficult—we have such different risk factors. Tumor size, follow-up therapies, cancer stage, and grade, play a role. Age is a factor. Young women who choose breast-conservation surgery and radiation have more local recurrences in the long run, than those who choose a single-sided mastectomy [6,11,46,118]. Your *margin status* (area free of cancer around the tissue removed) could impact every type of recurrence [49], although that is unknown before surgery. There is no exact consensus on what an appropriate cancer-free margin should be [168]. Different recommendations might be made if yours is less than a couple of millimeters, though generally, wide negative margins are better, even if the area receives radiation [168]. There is also the all-important *lymph node status* (if any of them have cancer). In some instances it might be possible to get a sense of lymph node involvement before surgery. Having such information would be helpful; aggressive surgeries provide limited benefit with an advanced breast cancer diagnosis.

Some experts believe that in time, 10% to 20% of patients will experience a local recurrence (on the treated side) with breast-conservation surgery, even after accounting for the benefits of radiation [49]. In December 2010, Dr. Judy Boughey, associate professor at the Mayo Clinic's Rochester, Minnesota, campus, was quoted on this topic. "If you get a lumpectomy, the risk of a local recurrence at *10 years* is 8% to 10%, and if you get a mastectomy, the risk is 2% to 4%" [118]. Your collective information will help you and your oncologists, as a team, explore your personal options and preferences.

The main advantage of CPM is the prevention of cancer on the opposite breast, although that risk is low for the majority of women. "On average, 5 prophylactic mastectomies would be needed to prevent the occurrence of one contralateral breast cancer." [163] The annual incidence (for most nonhereditary early stages) can be as low as .5% to .75% per year [121], or up to 1% annually [77], although the younger the woman at diagnosis, the more likely she is to have a *contralateral,* or an opposite, breast cancer episode. The possibility *continues* with time [158]. Women diagnosed in their 30s and 40s have a 15 to 20% lifetime risk, women diagnosed in their 50s have a 10% risk, and women in their 60s have a 5% risk [77]. In other words, older women do not benefit from CPM. They might not live long enough to develop a second breast cancer, including one on the opposite breast. Cancer on the opposite breast occurs (on average) to 15% of women with a history of breast cancer and no genetic predisposition [104]. Some studies have shown that 5% of women who choose a double mastectomy already have an *occult* (unknown) cancer on the opposite breast [63, 174]. CPM does *not* eliminate recurrences on the opposite side. It only diminishes the likelihood by 80 to 90% [12,110].

A friend of ours experienced the event. She chose a single-sided mastectomy with her first DCIS (or stage 0) breast cancer episode, and then developed cancer on her remaining breast 22 years later. Her second cancer infiltrated and breast-conservation surgery was recommended. She underwent radiation, endured chemotherapy, and she started an aromatase inhibitor. Her combined treatment is bound to be effective, but her 62-year-old body had a hard time.

Aside from age, other factors determine who might derive the greatest benefit from CPM. At the top of that list are patients with BRAC1 and BRAC2 genetic mutations [110], and then women with lobular breast cancer [121]. Women under the age of 49, who undergo CPM with their stage I or stage II hormone-receptor-negative breast cancer episode, might obtain a survival advantage [12], but most of us will not derive such a clear benefit. Some of us, who do not meet the mentioned criteria, might still derive some value from the surgery, although to a lesser extent. If we have a first-degree relative with breast cancer, if we have mammographic density, if our tumor biology suggests a higher recurrence rate, when our cancer infiltrates, or is in more than one location of the involved breast then, those factors either increase the likelihood of a second cancer, or can make follow-up screenings more challenging.

Both sides of this surgical argument might agree on one thing: those who face breast cancer again are bound to have a longer *disease-free period* (DFP, or time without cancer) with CPM, even if the mortality age from breast cancer is not delayed [70,132,163].

Interestingly, women are not always choosing CPM because they are at a higher risk of breast cancer on the opposite breast, or as a result of tumor characteristics [90]. Personal traits influence CPM decisions. Women who are young, white, and have a history of cancer choose it in higher numbers [158]. Those with high levels of education [77] or are married tend to be part of that group [35]. Other studies have found that, aside from family history, additional biopsies from MRI findings, failed attempts at breast-conservation surgery, and a plan to undergo immediate reconstruction were "predictors" for CPM [90].

It is clear that some of us do not *want* to keep our breast tissue under any circumstances. We do know that, for those of us with an early-stage diagnosis, breast-conservation surgery (along with other therapies) can give us a similar longevity benefit, and that proper surveillance catches most recurrences at an early stage. Most of us understand that most women will *not* have a recurrence with either method. Therefore, we might need to approach our surgical choice from a different perspective, a different set of questions, once we become informed.

So what should we ask ourselves if we are at a relatively early stage and we have the luxury to choose, what then? We can start by determining which surgical choice can give *each of us* the greatest sense of well-being for the rest of our life. Many women would never contemplate a double mastectomy, even if they have an elevated risk for the disease, and while some of us wish to avoid radiation and chemical therapies, others find they provide peace of mind. Stress worsens when therapy ends and follow-up appointments become infrequent. Which treatment do you fear most? Based on your *initial* surgical choice, and cancer stage, you might be able to avoid specific therapies.

Some patients decide against a mastectomy, and choose breast-conservation surgery after understanding the low recurrence rates [156], but detailed information and patient involvement might increase the mastectomy rate [35,83]. Some of those women cited "peace of mind" and "the wish to avoid radiation" as being more important than their ability to treat and keep their breast tissue [35]. A better understanding of the "late effects of breast irradiation" and the "oncologically safe" skin-sparing mastectomies (SSM) might be contributing to the higher mastectomy rate [8].

Avoiding therapies with breast-conservation surgery is not usually considered safe, although that too might change. Recent Oncotype DX technology might allow some women with DCIS (the earliest breast cancer stage) to bypass radiation. Though typically, with the exception of older women, radiation and anti-estrogen therapy (for hormone-sensitive breast cancers), are recommended to minimize DCIS recurrences [36,65]. After breast-conservation surgery annual mammograms should not be missed, although additional testing might be necessary. Obviously, ongoing screenings and anti-estrogen therapy are also needed after a single mastectomy.

While you are deciding keep in mind every treatment has the potential for complications, and no treatment offers guarantees. This is important. The main distinction, from a stress perspective, is uncertainty in different areas. With CPM there are more cosmetic and reconstructive issues, but less recurrence [61] and diagnostic screening concerns. On the other hand, "Women with DCIS treated with breast conservation continue to have diagnostic screenings and invasive procedures in the conserved breast over an extended period of time." [124]

To illustrate additional CPM benefits, I will continue to weave information with true survivor stories. I will start with the four of us diagnosed and treated for our early-stage breast cancers in the last four and a half years. We all had double mastectomies that could have been less aggressively treated. Each of us had a healthy breast removed, none of us had a genetic predisposition, and gladly, we all had acceptable cancer-free margins. We had different types of cancers, some aggressive, and we opted for different types of mastectomies and reconstructions. Our common factors were our early-stage diagnosis and our aggressive surgery, a combination that kept all of us from needing radiation. Even though three of us had hormone sensitive cancers, only one of us received a recommendation for hormone suppression therapy. We will all have annual follow-up visits, but not regular breast cancer screenings.

It would only be fair to admit our difficulties—those are usually the dissuading factors. All of our mastectomies and reconstructions took a while and had challenges. I had nerve damage; three of us had skin-healing challenges, and two of those required further interventions. I developed a capsular contracture, which required surgery, and two of us had muscular pain. All of those will show up on the complication statistics for contralateral prophylactic mastectomies, but all of us would do them again.

From a practical perspective, it might be necessary to consider finances. Health insurance policies and the coverage they provide vary. They do have to cover procedures that recreate symmetry, but the same does not apply to other aspects of treatment. They might have cancer-recurrence exclusions, or they might provide partial coverage. It won't be exact, but try to get a realistic short- and long-term out-of-pocket estimate from an insurance representative, for each and every therapy. Financial assistance is available for low-income patients, but obviously not everyone is eligible. With CPM more time away from work is required and reconstructions often involve other surgeries, although hopefully not on a regular basis. Breast-conservation surgery is typically followed by radiation and annual (or biannual) screenings. For women who need annual MRIs, have high insurance deductibles, high co-pays, or have lost or might lose insurance coverage, long-term surveillance could get expensive. A study presented at the 2010 ASCO Breast Cancer Symposium by investigators from the Mayo Clinic in Rochester, Minnesota, concluded that CPM might be cost-effective for those of us at average risk if we are also younger, assuming long-term surveillance costs are included [163]. Financial concerns might apply to the long-term cost of anti-estrogen therapy. In other words, the 20% to 40% of women who discontinue the therapy prematurely might have financial trepidations, not just side effects. If needed, prescription pharmaceuticals to lessen anti-estrogen therapy side effects also add to the cost, but share your concerns with health care providers before discontinuing any therapy prematurely; they might be able to help.

Financial considerations do not change our overall-survival statistics. Not unless important therapy is discontinued, or if missed screenings keep a recurrence from being diagnosed at a treatable stage. Hopefully financial concerns, including how difficult it can be to obtain or retain health insurance after a breast cancer diagnosis, will be lessened by health care reform in the USA.

Some of us want to avoid anti-estrogen therapy for other reasons. As I will explain later, I was afraid my family history of the potential complications, and my long-standing premenopausal and post-menopausal symptoms would be worsened by the therapy, a suspicion that was confirmed by my medical oncologist. I recall telling Sandy that I would try the therapy if it was strongly recommended, but if it added to my sense of imbalance as much as I feared, I would choose quality of life over length of life. I did not have to make the choice—my benefit would have been 2%. Thanks to my early-stage diagnosis, because I chose CPM, and as a result of my low Oncotype DX score, I got to avoid the therapy I feared most.

I am not against anti-estrogen therapy, not at all. In fact, I spent a long time convincing one survivor who chose breast-conservation surgery to start it, even though she was very hesitant. I emphasized that many women have no side effects, and that the pharmaceuticals can be *very* effective. Tamoxifen can reduce recurrences (including on the opposite breast) by as much as 50%, and aromatase inhibitors, which might be prescribed after menopause, could lessen the incidence by 75% [33]. I reinforced that not taking advantage of the therapy would keep her personal recurrence rate in the double digits. This was just my last treatment of choice.

The decision to decline anti-estrogen therapy needs to be discussed at length with appropriate specialists, although recommendations might vary. Even though the benefits are irrefutable for women who have estrogen-receptor positive (ER+) breast cancer, and either keep part of their breast tissue or have positive lymph nodes, not all of us have that certainty. If we choose CPM with a stage I diagnosis (which includes negative lymph nodes and acceptable cancer-free margins), or for DCIS treatment for estrogen-receptor positive (ER+) breast cancer, different recommendations seem to be the norm. Gene expression profiling, such as Oncotype DX and MammaPrint (which is FDA approved to analyze the aggressiveness of both hormone-receptor-positive and hormone-receptor-negative breast cancers at the time of biopsy) provide guidelines, but ultimately each of us, regardless of surgical choice, must determine which risks we are willing to take.

Even though my low Oncotype DX score is reassuring, the absence of anti-estrogen therapy lingers. It influences daily lifestyle choices. Four years later I still eat a well-balanced low-fat diet, I limit my alcohol intake, I exercise frequently, and I keep my weight in check. "On average, thinner breast cancer survivors live longer than heavier survivors," and survivors who exercise four to nine hours weekly might reduce the likelihood of a recurrence by 20% to 40% [94].

The length of a study, the criteria to analyze the data, and the ages of the participants can all vary, but if you choose to tackle the difficult task of deciphering statistics, you should ask yourself these questions. Do the recurrence statistics include all possible events on breast tissue, including on the opposite breast? How long is the study? Does it provide a recurrence breakdown by breast cancer stage? Is yours well represented? Studies on CPM might include various stages, up to stage III [174]. For obvious reasons, different stages have a different long-term prognosis. So many variables, including personal cancer data, might explain why typically neither long-term recurrence statistics, nor long-term survival statistics, are available by stage or by surgical choice. "Cancer survival is typically reported in terms of five-year survival." [22]

To further complicate matters, studies, experts, and even we the patients disagree with each other on many breast cancer topics, including on screening recommendations, but more on that later. Try to become familiar with different angles before forming an opinion. For example, while most see non-hereditary, early-stage local recurrences as low, some of us don't see them that way. If a study is large and long term, then those up-to-date findings can be considered more reliable. Sorting recurrence information is not only difficult, reported outcomes might be influenced by personal biases [129]. In other words, research but consider different perspectives before making a decision.

Numbers should not be the only consideration. Long-term contentment with *any* choice seems to be higher for patients who choose for themselves [83]. Although, it is hard to know how many women wish they had chosen more aggressive surgery. Surgical regret surveys are typically done on women who choose some type of mastectomy—not on those who keep their healthy breast tissue. And yet, one small study showed that surgical regret among young breast-conservation patients might not be uncommon [51]. That might explain why I have met six women who had breast-conservation surgery, and who wish they had chosen a bilateral mastectomy when they were first diagnosed. I will recount the story of four, although again, keep in mind they don't necessarily represent their surgical counterparts.

The first woman has been experiencing joint pain and severe hot flashes from her anti-estrogen therapy for years. Since the side effects did not respond to traditional methods, both affected her quality of life and her sleep. She wonders if a double mastectomy would have kept her from requiring the therapy, because she too had negative lymph nodes.

The second woman was waiting for the result of her second biopsy on the opposite breast, 10 years after her breast-conservation-surgery treatment. In retrospect, she would have preferred CPM to avoid the stress from the annual screenings, and the anxiety from the biopsies. She might have still needed biopsies with a double mastectomy—they just would have been less likely.

The third survivor had a recurrence on her breast-conservation side, but after the necessary mastectomy, her previously radiated tissue could not handle the reconstruction-expansion attempt. Tissue-graft reconstructions are her only option and she is hesitant. They are much bigger surgeries. She had considered herself cured. Her initial recurrence statistics were at 3%, and two years before she finished 5 years of anti-estrogen therapy. This time she came close to needing chemotherapy, and an aromatase inhibitor was recommended.

The fourth woman had painful radiation scarring and felt disfigured from skin changes and asymmetry after breast-conservation surgery. She often wondered if a double mastectomy, either skin or nipple sparing, along with reconstruction and without radiation, might have prevented some of those problems. A few years later she chose CPM after a local recurrence. Due to her previous radiation she opted for a graft reconstruction. Unfortunately she experienced serious complications and the graft did not take.

Again, local recurrences can still happen after CPM—some breast tissue inevitably remains. They are just less likely, or they might happen later. Local recurrences are simply higher with breast-conservation surgeries [46]. The mentioned recurrences affected 10-year or 5-year recurrence statistics, not overall-survival statistics (OS).

Reconstructive hurdles are also possible when a *first* breast cancer episode is followed by CPM. The difference is that without radiation the chances are diminished, the likelihood of symmetry is greater, and the reconstructive options can be broader. In 2010 Moffit Cancer Center launched a clinical trial for women interested in either a nipple-sparing mastectomy or a skin-sparing mastectomy, assuming they are at an early enough stage. Unfortunately, those with previous radiation or surgery in proximity to the nipple are not eligible [97].

And yet, I did not choose a bilateral mastectomy because of cosmetic benefits, due to financial concerns, or as a result of recurrence worries. In *my* opinion this was the gentlest preference, given the options. I chose to remove *only* the tissue that already was or was most likely to become hostile, rather than attack parts of my body that were not yet a threat and would probably never become one. I was also thinking about long-term treatment options. The three of us, who initially chose CPM and had never been treated for breast cancer, still have our radiation card safely tucked away in our back pocket for a rainy day. We can still rely on this trump card if we have a recurrence (or a new cancer) on our affected side. Usually no one area can receive radiation twice.

Research your options, ask, and ask again. Discuss your cosmetic concerns with a couple of plastic surgeons and request visuals of realistic outcomes. You too might be amazed at how cosmetic outcomes can be improved after every type of surgery. If mastectomy is a consideration, then you might want to find out if you are a candidate for either a skin or a nipple sparing procedure, although look for a surgeon who frequently performs those surgeries. If finances are an issue, the American Cancer Society provides assistance for out of town consultations and care to those who qualify. If you are contemplating CPM, it might be reassuring to know that in the long run, 70% to 90% of us who choose to have our healthy breast removed do not regret our decision [57,61,64].

Regardless of what you choose, take the time to determine what is right for *you*. I know how difficult it is to make your surgical selection. You are living through some of the most stressful days of your life, while having the complication, the recurrence, and the overall survival Russian roulette guns at your temple.

$$\text{\textcircled{$\mathscr{L}$}}$$

FAMILY COPING & SURGERY PREPARATIONS

Once all of the surgery decisions were made, our focus shifted to the home front. We tried to keep ourselves from panicking into the future, although that was easier said than done. It seemed important to recognize what was still good in our lives, even though our world had been turned upside down. Staying positive for my family did not come naturally. I had to work at it. When I was having trouble I asked myself these questions: How can I remain in a state of gratitude? Is it possible to learn from this situation? What is the best example for our children?

We attempted to lower our stress by limiting phone conversations. Speaking on the phone, giving bad news, and sensing the stress of our loved ones in their voices and in their silences increased our anxiety. Since not all conversations could be avoided we opted to speak on the phone when our children were at school, or at least in another room.

If over communication causes stress, then I suggest you limit it. This is one thing you can control. By skipping frequent cancer explanations we got to focus on our children, on decision making, on researching, and on listening to what felt right. To limit socialization I recommend you ask key people in your social and family circles to act as communicators. I encouraged our friends to pass the news along, but I did not want phone calls. People were able to reach out with cards, emails, and through our blog.

Our favorite coping skill became valuable for months. Since rare moments of normality would often manifest themselves during meals, we tried to continue our routine of eating dinner together on most nights without electronic interruptions. We also resorted to our typical joking. Behaving normally was not easy, but we persevered. As we did, we were rewarded with the ability to comfortably move from one stressful situation to another. Humor kept our teenagers wanting to come home. Without it, they might have stayed away. In time we received the unexpected gift of stronger family bonds, which only continued over time. Initially those glimpses of normality were only possible between the four of us. Many people felt our humor was out of place; they were not sure how to approach us or how to respond. Eventually, and by example, we convinced them otherwise.

A parent's cancer diagnosis presents older teens with interesting dilemmas. At an age when they usually take their parents for granted, they are forced to contemplate their parent's mortality. My teenagers were old enough to understand the magnitude of a cancer diagnosis, although not experienced enough to have the coping skills. They needed space but not too much. Even though they had no choice, our teens would have preferred to avoid cancer discussions. They did not know how to ask questions, but they had many. Just as they were starting to explore their independence, they felt the need to stay by our side.

Our adolescents needed honest information as it became available, but we tried to focus on the positive aspects of each new development. From their body language, tone of voice, or from any atypical behaviors, I tried to read what they were experiencing or needed. Sometimes by simply making time to be with them, unexpected, in-depth conversations would take place. During those precious opportunities I helped them cope with their conflicting emotions. I gave them permission to be joyful and encouraged them to stay focused on their typical priorities. I explained the importance of not suppressing their fears and sorrows, while reassuring them I could handle them if they wanted to explore them with me.

Trying to balance our family's emotional tone gave me a sense of control in the midst of so much uncertainty. We did discuss difficult subjects, but for the sake of our collective sanity those could not be the norm. I tried to keep my emotions on the back burner. On occasion I asked the "why me?" question—I just tried not to stay there for long; it was too stressful to contemplate at the time. There would be plenty of time for that type of soul searching later.

My extended family got together to show their support. That was amazing. Getting all of us together is difficult under the best of circumstances. Our reunions can include over 20 people, and some of our children are grown and busy with their own lives. At the time we were scattered throughout the state, out of the state, and out of the country. The gesture proved that I am fortunate to have an amazing family, not just during difficult times, all of the time.

I tried to prepare for the road ahead with books and information, although I found very few resources that addressed my middle station in life. From the quest I learned that older women are less likely to undergo reconstructions. Some books and resources focus on younger survivors, who have specific priorities. They are trying to identify possible genetic risks, and by extension early breast cancer screening awareness among their peers. Young survivors often need to become familiar with treatment-induced fertility issues. While they undergo multiple breast cancer therapies, they also have to juggle work and the parenting of young children. As I read about the growing number of young women affected by breast cancer, I realized that those stressors would be far more daunting.

I also searched for books containing a mix of practical information and family coping examples, except I realized that most breast cancer books are focused on providing medical information, coping skills, general suggestions, or personal stories. I wanted a *mix* of those with clear teen scenarios. In many respects including this one, I wound up writing the book I was hoping to find.

There were practical matters to attend to as well. It was important to prepare our house, our cars, and our supplies. We bought as many nonperishable items as budget and space allowed, we arranged car pools, and we filled prescriptions. We tuned up our cars, did necessary home maintenance, and we paid bills in advance. We should have positioned frequently used items at a lower level in our closet and in the kitchen. Reaching in those areas became particularly challenging for a long time.

As we prepared it became clear how little Sandy understood about our paperwork and about the ins and outs of running our house. Although he refused to get too involved, he expressed I would be well soon enough. He could not have known that he would become familiar with nearly every one of those tasks; I would be unable to perform many of them for years. From his dismissive demeanor I sensed that his hesitation was on a bigger scale—my absence on any level was frightening. He was not prepared to contemplate the possibility.

Part Two

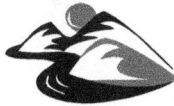

Communication

The activity of conveying meaningful information as by speech, signals, writing, or behavior. Derived from the Latin word "communis", meaning to share. It requires a sender, a message, and an intended recipient.

(Wikipedia)

THE BLOG:
DOUBLE MASTECTOMY & RECONSTRUCTION
March 22nd 2009 - June 24th 2009

"Self-expression must pass into communication for its fulfillment."
— Pearl S. Buck

"Communication is a continual balancing act, juggling the conflicting needs for intimacy and independence. To survive in the world, we have to act in concert with others, but to survive as ourselves, rather than simply as cogs in a wheel, we have to act alone."

— Deborah Tannen

My external composure seldom betrayed the storm raging within. How could I relay the sensation of being at the edge of a precipice? Would it have served a purpose? What made it possible to keep functioning for weeks with a feeling of impending doom? Was I sensing the difficulties that would linger far longer than anticipated?

Distractions could no longer suppress my anxiety. The house was impeccable, there was nothing else to research, we had supplies to last us for weeks, and my bags were packed. I did not venture outside. I did not want to see concern in familiar eyes. I was afraid conversations about the impending ordeal would tip me over the edge prematurely. By extension, the phone did not seem like a friendly instrument. The fear I was trying to avoid had seeped into every voice, although to my dismay the phone would not stop ringing. One survivor described this extreme level of stress as "an out-of-body experience." The body moves but the mind is elsewhere. Another survivor explained how, even though the world continued to revolve, before her surgery her life had come to a standstill.

And yet, we could not ignore our responsibility—we had to communicate with the outside world. When he suggested we set up a blog, Neil's electronic ingenuity solved the dilemma. He was right. You might want to consider this communication method if you are feeling overwhelmed. With just one update every few days blogging kept many informed at their convenience. We were able to avoid individual responses, as would have been the case with either emails or with phone calls. Setting up a blog gave my worried son something concrete to do, and Nicole derived a similar benefit by typing entries.

Our blog was open from the day before my double mastectomy until a week after my first reconstructive surgery, when most of my breast cancer journey should have ended. That was not the case. I developed a capsular contracture and I was asymmetric. I was not interested in grieving my setback in a public forum, but within days I began to miss the documentation. In time blogging led to journaling and that led to more writing, although obviously, I was unaware of long-term hidden agendas when we began communicating through this unfamiliar, though user friendly medium.

Dear reader: for the sake of clarity some entries were deleted, others were slightly altered, and I added remarks. Blog entries are in *non-bold italics* and the few breast-cancer related responses I kept are and in ***bold italics***.

March 21st

I would like to apologize to those of you who are receiving our news in this manner. You are important to us, but time is suddenly a precious commodity. We have a lot to do under a lot of stress, and speaking about this is very hard. If you have already heard our sad news, please be patient as I reiterate for the rest.

The short version is that approximately a month ago I was diagnosed with breast cancer. After careful consideration, and because the cancer was not easily diagnosed, I've chosen a double mastectomy as my treatment. This is undoubtedly the right choice for me, and even though the decision seems drastic, I am at peace with my decision. The reconstruction will take several weeks and further treatment will depend on surgical findings, but we will cross that bridge when we get there.

I am already indebted to many, starting with my extended family for the impromptu get-together—I feel your love. To my daughter, Nicole, thank you for your amazingness! To Neil, thanks for the hours you spent setting this up! Sandy, thank you for being perfectly supportive, I couldn't ask for more. Mom, knowing I can count on you unconditionally is priceless but you might regret it!

We are fortunate to have such a support system in you, our family and friends. We will be relying on many of you in the coming weeks. Please forward this link to those we know in common. To all who have sent cards, texts, and emails, you make me feel loved. Andrew, Mela, and my book club girls, your book timing is impeccable. Diane, thank you for all the driving, the extra rest has made a huge difference. Shelley and Debbie, thank you for organizing meals, they will undoubtedly come in handy. Like I said, the phone is hard and time consuming, especially since most of our focus is on the kids. We want them to feel a sense of continuity, and yes, also joy! So far, we have accomplished our goal.

The first paragraph in <u>A Tale of Two Cities</u> *by Charles Dickens illustrates our roller coaster over the last few weeks, and the same will undoubtedly apply to the ones to come as well. "It was the best of times, it was the worst of times ... it was the epoch of belief, it was the epoch of incredulity, it was the season of Light, it was the season of Darkness, it was the ... winter of despair..." Please know that your loving support helps to dissipate the darkness. — Jenny*

P.S. ***PROPS TO THE BEST DAUGHTER EVER, NICOLE CLAIRE GLIKIN, FOR TYPING THIS FOR ME! :) Oh yeah, Neil also helped a little.

The night before surgery we said goodbye to my intact body with a tear laced intimate expression. The next morning I too bid farewell, although I also wondered what reflection I would find the next time I stood in front of my old mirror.

◈

SURGERY

We arrived at the hospital with plenty of time to spare. With the planned sentinel lymph node biopsy (SLND), only a few lymph nodes would be removed to check for cancer. But the dye, which was injected in several locations without an anesthetic, had to be in place an hour before the surgery. The ensuing discomfort raised my anxiety level, though I was still determined to undergo the planned procedure.

Cancer's footprint felt very large that day. Dozens would arrive later that day, and thousands were doing the same thing in other facilities, a dreadful routine that repeats itself on any given day. I wondered who was familiar with the ominous procedure and how they were managing. None of us spoke about our stress. At least on the surface we appeared composed. My apprehension was lessened by our rabbi's blessing and reassurance. He shared that most of the women he has seen in a similar circumstance are not only surviving after their breast cancer ordeals, they are thriving.

We are all different and you might want to make different choices, but before surgery I did not want to be with anyone other than our children, Sandy, and our rabbi. I was not sure how I was going to respond, though in the end I managed to look very composed, even when the surgical gurney came to carry me into the operating room. At that point I was already wearing my large blue hospital gown, which so cleverly disguised the various markings that had been strategically drawn all over my chest.

March 23rd

Hello all. I bring positive news. Jenny is moving from the OR to the recovery room as I type this. The surgeons report that all of the lymph nodes are negative (meaning there has been no spread of the cancer). The breast tissue removal and the first stage of the reconstruction have also gone well. We expect to be released from the hospital in the morning.

Your faithful blogger, Sandy

Sandy,

Just catching up with my emails—this is a little high tech for me :) Absolutely wonderful news that all nodes are clear and that Jenny's surgery has gone well! What a relief that must be for you (I know the feeling, brother—been there, done that). Let Jenny know that we have been thinking of her and praying for her (as well as for you and your family). Let us know how we can make your life easier. Hope all continues to go well. See you around the shop sometime soon.

— B.

A Blog Entry by Neil (my 17-year-old son)

March 23rd—After the Visit ... Sleep Well.

I saw my mother again this evening following her operation. Her arrival to the hospital room had been a bit delayed, as she had been experiencing considerable pain in the recovery room. Though we had all (my father, sister, grandmother, and I) been uplifted upon hearing the good news from the surgery as mentioned in the previous post, her condition was still a difficult sight to bear. She was pale, barely conscious, and clearly in pain. Seeing her was especially difficult for my sister, as well as for my grandmother.

My mother's condition improved considerably after receiving some morphine. She was interacting with us and even comforting us. I no longer needed comfort. I could see that inside she remained strong. She was fighting through her pain so that she could show us she would be okay. Physically weak as she may have been, tonight she was emotionally and spiritually as strong as ever. Even in her pain she could not stop caring for us. She felt it necessary to express her gratitude, and she was concerned about our schoolwork. Indeed, I no longer needed comfort. It is clearer than ever that my mother has the strength to fight through the toughest of times for herself and for all of us. I hope her recovery will be speedy.

At the moment she remains in the hospital to (attempt to) sleep for the night with my father at her side. Hopefully she will return home tomorrow. And again, we are all so glad the surgery went as well as it possibly could.

I love you mom — Neil

Mom seeing you tonight was just about the hardest thing ever ... I know that it will get better though. I can't wait for you to come home. I miss you — Nicole

I wanted Neil and Nicole at the hospital when I came out of surgery. I did not want to sugarcoat my cancer. I sensed that at 15 and 17 years old they were old enough to handle the experience. I also wanted them to support each other during the waiting, which would not have been easier at home without their father.

Although I had no idea how difficult it would be for them to see me after surgery, I did not expect to be so uncomfortable. And yet, if I had to do it again I would offer them the same opportunity. They now know healing can take place from that level of discomfort. They also got to experience the importance of family support during a stressful time, which will undoubtedly serve them well in the future.

The level of pain I was experiencing was surprising. I knew most patients are not as uncomfortable. I had been under a misconception; I thought delivering three babies without sedatives or epidurals had prepared me, but that was not the case. The pain, the anesthesia, and the Morphine made it difficult to keep my eyes open long enough to see my mother, Sandy, Neil, and Nicole. They had been there four hours beyond what had been anticipated. I was glad to see them, even though we were basically in parallel universes. I was alone in a terrible place, and I was trying to crawl my way out of it.

⸎

GOING HOME

March 24th

After a pain-filled evening and a long night, the warm Florida sun rose to find Jenny feeling a bit better. Still sore and tired, but able to use oral medications rather than IV ones (directly into the bloodstream) to control the pain. After a visit by the physical therapist, a lap around the ward, followed by a needed rest and a second attempt at hospital food, it was time to go home. We arrived at 6 PM and were soon greeted by some of our wonderful neighbors and a complete dinner for all of us, confirmation that coming home was the right thing to do. We are looking forward to getting some sleep and anticipate continued improvement in the morning.

We appreciate all of the comments, positive thoughts, and prayers. This is just the beginning of a long road and there's no turning back. Some of the pavement will not be smooth, but we are heading in the right direction.

Your blogmeister — Sandy

A lot changed during my short departure. In the hospital being a patient felt normal, and having people care for me could even be considered routine, but once

I crossed the threshold into our home being a patient felt altogether wrong. The very place I had called home for 14 years, where I had taken care of my family, entertained our friends, prepared most meals, and kept track of nearly every coming and going, that place became impossible to navigate without assistance for several weeks.

All of that was unexpected. I had not read anywhere that getting up, turning in bed, or lifting a glass of water would be so difficult. It was impossible to open a door, reach for anything above my waist, or in any direction other than in front of me. These restrictions frightened me; I knew they were atypical, but I did not know how long they would last. It was humbling to feel so weak, especially since just the day before I had been so strong and in control of my body.

I had to revise my definition of *normal.* Comparing the new state of affairs with the old was simply too depressing. I tried to remain focused. Unbeknownst to them, Neil and Nicole were making mental notes that would be retrieved in their future time of need. I set out to show them it was okay for the nurturer to be nurtured, and for the child to temporarily switch roles with the parent. Although to accomplish those goals, and for the sake of sanity, I needed to be open to receiving help, resting, and giving up my title of being in charge. None of that was easy—being in control had nearly defined me just the day before. Even so, there was no time for self-pity. I had to rise to the occasion, this was the real deal—it was show time.

❧

INCISION CARE, PAIN & ANXIETY MANAGEMENT

As many of you already know, looking at our chest after surgery is very difficult. For the first few days I was in too much discomfort and under too much stress to contemplate the possibility. While Sandy emptied the drains and checked my wounds, my focus was on avoiding the mirror. Everything felt strange—quite literally. My entire chest, underarms, and upper arms were numb to the touch, just like my face had felt after being anesthetized at the dentist's office. And yet, as if it was some kind of a sick joke, I still managed to have enough internal sensation to experience pain—a lot of it.

Playing music and timing the unpleasant activities made a difference. I could not change my dressings first thing in the morning; it was a hard way to start the day. I could not be too tired—that made it harder to bear. I took a pain pill 30 minutes before the unpleasant activity, but above all, deep breathing techniques eased my anxiety.

I would like to suggest the very things I did to minimize the likelihood of an infection. Aside from making sure my hands were clean, I used disposable gloves. I got individually wrapped alcohol wipes for cleaning the drain tips, before and after emptying the drainage. I used disposable plastic medicine cups, and to dry the incisions, I opted for disposable sterile gauze instead of a towel. Prior to showering I left the necessary items ready, including the chart and the pencil to document the drainage.

It seemed necessary to cover the incisions, even though many doctors prefer they remain uncovered. The edge of the bra against the incisions was painful, but not as uncomfortable as the lack of support. Once I got my plastic surgeon's approval, I covered the incisions with *Telfa* gauze, which does not adhere to the skin and is painless to remove. I chose paper tape. It too is easier to peel, but I did not apply it directly on the incisions; to avoid separating the edges, I placed it horizontally above and below. Besides, to heal, incisions need air. The light covering protected the incisions, kept fabric from rubbing against them, and kept them cleaner than they would have been otherwise. The process was lengthy, but it minimized the discomfort. I tried to remain detached, but that didn't always work as well as I hoped.

Even the skin on my chest needed special treatment. In order to prevent further dryness or irritation, I had to avoid lotions with perfumes or alcohol. Although, my plastic surgeon explained that to prevent infections, creams should be kept away from *fresh* incisions. A heavy antibacterial ointment was necessary for weeks on both nipples; all of that skin turned black—it looked like I was going to lose it all. To reassure me my plastic surgeon reminded me that skin heals from the inside out. Luckily it did, after several long, stressful weeks. Since I wanted to keep those areas moist, and to prevent the ointment from adhering to my clothing, I made sure those areas were also covered with the non-adhesive gauze. The mentioned items should be available in drug stores.

I took narcotics as often as I was allowed for the first four days, but I then got severely constipated. I was having trouble eating and hydrating, which nearly prompted a trip to the emergency room. The scenario can be avoided. My nursing experience had taught me the importance of laxatives, or at least stool softeners along with narcotics, but in the midst of so much pain and stress my judgment seemed absent. When I stopped the narcotics I realized that over-the-counter pain relievers worked just as well, or perhaps better said, just as poorly. There was a good reason for the limited benefit: narcotics are often ineffective for nerve pain [142]. A muscle relaxant was the next recommendation, unfortunately those made me nauseous and their benefit was minimal.

∞

SHORT-LIVED PROGRESS

March 27th

Hello blogosphere. We may have turned the corner. Jenny got up this morning feeling less pain, and even helped to prepare Nicole for school at 6:30 (even though she did not need to, obviously). She spent less time sleeping and is eating more (many thanks to Nana Elsa and our generous neighbors). When Nicole came home from school today, her comment was "mom looks like mom." She got dressed, put on makeup and earrings, and even felt well enough to take a car ride. More tellingly she picked up her books, which are her passion. Neil is out of town with his school band. He will be stunned to see Jenny's progress when he gets back on Sunday. Certainly there will still be hard days, but today was nothing short of a pleasure. I've gone back to work, but she remains in the competent hands of her mother. We are lucky to have her around. Without her this would have been harder for both of us.

To those of you with whom I haven't spoken for much too long (you know who you are), thanks for the calls. I won't stay away again.

— Sanford Glikinblogger

You and Sandy and the kids have been in our hearts all week. Glad to know that each day is a little better. This week marks ten years for me as a breast cancer survivor. Even though my experience was not as trying as yours, I can say the tremendous love and strength you feel as a family now, will only become more so. Thank you for keeping us updated. You are in our hearts each day. Be kind and patient with yourself ...

Love, S & G

Unlike most women, my sense of improvement would be short lived. Gladly, the majority of survivors do not regress as I did. It was difficult to imagine how my reconstruction would amount to anything that resembled normality. The skin throughout my chest was bruised, my nipples looked like they had lost their blood supply, and the incisions were quite noticeable. Fortunately all improved with time. If you find yourself in this situation, keep in mind that reconstructions take time. It might be several weeks or months before your reconstruction looks as well as it is going to look.

ꟾꟾꟾ

No More Drains! An Entry by Nicole (My 15-Year-Old Daughter)

March 31st

Today my madre got her drains snatched (that's a good thing). She can now wear shirts that button in the front, and my father ironed them before she went out.

Now, if you think she is doing everything for herself, you're wrong :) I am doing the dishes, taking the dog out, reaching everything that she can't and MORE!! She also cooked dinner tonight, but not really, I pretty much had to do it all. But since she claims she made it, I'm gonna go along with it. Meanwhile, her husband is doing everything else including working. What a handsome studly guy ... ha ha—not. Neil has also suffered. He lost his lamp to mom, is organizing his own carpool, has to do his own laundry, and has even helped in the kitchen, which is VERY rare for him, not for me! In other words, she's got it made. Isn't she so lucky??? Oh yeah, I forgot one thing. Thanks for the amazing food, especially the ziti, lasagna, and the coffee cake. You know who you are, keep it comin! :)

My dad says: "have your teenager translate, I can't help." I don't know why he is saying that. No translation is needed. I apologize on behalf of his weirdness :) — NICOLE

ꟾꟾꟾ

Dressing after Breast Cancer Surgery & Beyond

Inadequate clothing coverage increased my stress levels and made me self-conscious when I went out. I tried to anticipate my needs, but I did it poorly.

Bra sizes, or even comfortable ones, were impossible to predict. Although buying extra bra extenders at a fabric store, and removing wires through a small opening minimized the discomfort. I wish I had known about bras intended for mastectomy patients who do not reconstruct; they have less lace and softer fabrics. They can be worn without the prosthetic insert, with only one insert, or with different size inserts. They could have made a difference during the height of my discomfort or when I experienced asymmetry. Sports bras that do not open are downright impossible for many of us on a permanent basis. Several women have shared that finding comfortable bras can be a long-term challenge. The process involves a lot of trial and error, as well as expense. Some of us find it necessary to avoid seams in a particular area and that even lace can hurt. With time—the ultimate healer—and with proper scar tissue management some discomfort can be lessened. Massages to minimize scar tissue should only be attempted once your surgeon deems it safe. I will share what I learned about scar tissue management later.

Some purchases were not useful. Tight skin and unstretched muscles kept the expanders right below my clavicles for weeks and ruled out scooped-neck shirts. During that time I lived in zip-up terrycloth robes, one of my best purchases. Aside from how easy they were to put on, the thickness of the fabric concealed the irregular lumps on my chest, the bulk of the drains, and the lengthy tubing quite well. Our friend Shelley helped. She let me borrow all of her long, front-button-up shirts, and those became my primary wardrobe for several weeks.

From the perspective of discreetness, one survivor explained that she resorts to "distracting wear." Prints, sequins, and even jewelry can draw attention away from our chest area, which much to our dismay becomes an area of interest on an ongoing basis.

⚮

CHEMOTHERAPY CONSIDERATION

April 6th

With the help of my secretary Nicole, I will provide an update. Even if they are only temporary, no shortcuts are allowed during this process. The pain continues, asthma has been thrown in for excitement, and at a doctor's appointment I received concerning news. My "tissue report" (the pathology on the tissue removed in surgery) explained why a double mastectomy was my first choice, instead of the usual lumpectomy, for what appeared to be a small, localized lesion. Upon microscopic examination the tumor was not only larger, the disease had spread through several milk ducts.

This development suddenly makes me a candidate for chemotherapy. However, in case you are wondering where all of that cancer fundraising goes, let me give you an example. Even as we speak my tumor is undergoing Oncotype DX gene evaluation. Once I got over the shock, I am finding the ability to obtain such information reassuring. The findings will help determine the future likelihood of spread and if chemotherapy is needed.

Otherwise I am progressing well. Most of the skin has adhered to my pectoral muscles, and reconstructive efforts will resume next week. As recommended by my oncologist's office, I started treatment with an acupuncturist to reduce pain. I would also like to avoid steroids, which I've always needed during asthma episodes. On the upside, I am moving a little better, I can shower alone, and I got my (amazing) hairdresser Nicole to straighten my hair. We've had some delicious meals, and the beauty of our home has been enhanced in nearly every room with beautiful cards and flowers. THANKS!!! :D (That's a smiley face by the way).

I look forward to a summer of enjoying my family (especially Nicole). These past months have been trying—we need and deserve a break. We will be present at Andrew's master's degree graduation, even though I am still recovering. We don't want to miss his important milestone. For now, I will focus on the healing that has taken place, and I will try to appreciate that the right choices were made.

— Jenny (well technically Nicole, but whateverrr)

The tissue report was concerning. I tried to focus on what had gone well, though even then I felt completely overwhelmed. Coping moment to moment was the only way I could get by. I will again rely on this coping skill, it was that effective.

Acupuncture did not relieve my discomfort. If you are considering acupuncture, take the time to find a very experienced licensed practitioner. That is what I did at a later date with undeniable results.

PAIN LIMITING MOBILITY

April 13th

Pain seems to interfere with everything. My driving privileges will soon be restored, but I will not be ready. The back of my left arm and underarm are numb, I am very weak, I am shaky from the steroids, and my pectoral muscles are once again incredibly tight, painful, and guarded. I never realized that the pectoral muscles are involved in so many movements including holding a pen, that a jug of lemonade could feel so heavy, and that opening a bathroom door could prove impossible. During periods of increased pain even a deep breath hurts. I instinctually limit mobility for the sake of comfort. Luckily I have meditated for a number of years. During those blissful moments all pain is lifted and I am able to regain my perspective.

My strategy, since I must always have one, is to slow down the reconstructive process. I want to give my skin and my pectoral muscles a chance to stretch slowly to lessen the discomfort. To maximize my traveling comfort, the week before Andrew's graduation I will avoid a fill. After that I will be able to use our pool. Our backyard will become a spa! I believe water will help restore my strength. I can almost taste it.

I am beginning to see why these experiences are so life changing. Living without pain will never be taken for granted again. So many lessons ...

— Jenny

I could not understand why I was experiencing more pain than most mastectomy patients. I assumed that surgical trauma and swelling were the culprits, what I did not know was that nerve damage and limited shoulder motion were also contributing. Muscle spasms were part of the mix. I thought heat might help those spasms, but my plastic surgeon warned me. Due to the chest numbness, he was afraid I would suffer from either heat or ice burns, as others have done. The waves of discomfort were eased by gentle self-massages and with relaxation techniques, particularly after saline was added into the expanders.

☙

A Setback with a Parental Silver Lining

Shortly after we typed that blog entry my breathing, strength, and my mobility worsened, as the asthma progressed. Even walking around the block became impossible for weeks. The coughing increased the chest tightness, the high steroid dose made it impossible to sleep, and the vicious cycle was aggravated by the possibility of chemotherapy. I've often wondered if my recovery would have continued without the additional pain and the inopportune shortness of breath. As expected, I became depressed and withdrew from most human contact.

My boys felt helpless, but despite the multiple challenges, the period provided an opportunity to bond with the only person who understood what I needed—my daughter. She stayed with me from the time she came home from school to nearly the moment she went to sleep. She did her school work by my side, we watched TV together, and we listened to music together. At times she tried to make me laugh, she knew when to be silent, and she even knew when to remind me the surgery was a success. How could she have known that all I really needed was moral support? Not even I understood the obvious need. Her womanly intuition could have played a role—she was so close to being a woman. Her affection and approach wise beyond her 15 years floored me. I will always be grateful for those challenging weeks.

Encourage your teenagers to help or spend as much time with you as they are willing. Those occasions can be golden opportunities. By allowing my daughter to be so involved I got to know her better. Since I had her full attention I became familiar with her music, I watched her favorite shows, and I heard more about her friends. The time together provided a distraction and improved our relationship. Much to my surprise she matured from our difficult, shared experience. She was watching how I coped with the situation moment to moment and made me rise to the occasion—I faked it until I made it.

⸎

Temporary Progress—Again

April 29th

The healing Florida sun has improved my sense of well-being. As asthma releases its clutch, the familiar joy for the ability to breath with ease comes over me, although the gratitude is perhaps a little more evident this time around. Having smaller saline injections has made the waves of pain less frequent and intense. I only have two more over the next three weeks. Then a month later, possibly around mid-June, I will return to surgery for the permanent implants.

I regained a little sensation to the upper part of my left arm and apparently this is lucky at four weeks—it can take two years. Full range of motion and strength still elude me, but there is joy in mundane tasks, even if they are accomplished with two hands, rather than one. Lifting a skillet, reaching the bottom of the washing machine, and opening a blind are all symbolic of increased mobility, strength and independence.

I have not spoken about Sandy but I really must. He has stepped up to the plate with poise, willingness, love, and with his peculiar sense of humor that keeps us grounded. I cannot imagine what this experience would be like without a partner like him. Our children are lucky to have such a positive day-to-day example during difficult times. I can only hope they will be as lucky in their relationships, as I have been with him.

There is a wonderful "new normal" for activities such as grocery shopping. Since I can go out but not yet reach, lift, or drive as well as I should, the outing is now performed with a friend, which is perhaps how it should always be conducted. Food gathering, along with companionship, conversation, and then wrapped up with a hug is very pleasant.

It really does take a village, and mine is very large and kind.

Thank you! — Jenny

After my surgery people from various social circles were suddenly driving our children, bringing meals, sending gifts, walking our dog Magic, taking me to medical appointments, and to the grocery store. I was overwhelmed. Prior to cancer I felt like I was not living up to my expectations, or to those of my loved ones. After cancer I began to reconsider those sentiments, and you might want to contemplate doing the same. *If so many people feel that you are special enough to deserve so much attention, then perhaps it is time for you to start believing it as well.* The unexpected kindness moved me, made me feel loved, and changed me one kindness at a time. Even though I did not think it possible, the level of self-acceptance that I had been seeking most of my life began to emerge.

As usual steroids lessened the asthma symptoms, but when they were discontinued the muscular pain increased with a vengeance. Those symptoms—along with continued tiredness and weakness—were worsened by an endocrine imbalance that was probably present before cancer. The imbalance could have been exacerbated by the combination of surgery, pain, stress, and by the long course of steroids to treat the asthma. Endocrine issues, along with the nerve damage, kept my muscles painfully weak for a very long time. The resulting complications (including muscular asymmetries) would fluctuate between slight improvement and lost ground over the next year and a half.

Perhaps at the time ignorance was bliss, but if I had known what was going on, and to keep the problems from progressing as much as they did, I would have focused on very specific movements and complementary approaches. I would have also addressed the endocrine problems, which became unavoidable later, but doing so finally reduced my fatigue and made my muscular healing possible.

◈

A MUCH-NEEDED RECONSTRUCTION REPRIEVE

May 5th

Everything was perfect at Andrew's graduation and with some undeniable parallels. Spring was in the air in New England, as well as within me, and Andrew is experiencing a new beginning, as are we. We are so proud of him! Having his parents, his stepparents, our cousin Ira, and his lovely wife Yvonne there was amazing. As if that was not enough, we also got to stay in Boston to see our cousin Mona and her family. Wow!

Soon I will be done with saline fills. For a natural look my plastic surgeon is trying to overstretch the pectoral muscle 10 to 20% beyond the ultimate size. I am encouraged—the outcome might be better than I had expected. I might look and feel very normal.

There is no word yet on the Oncotype DX, but I do have an appointment with the oncologist in two weeks. Perhaps the results will be ready by then. Somehow I am not as worried. I KNOW I will be fine with or without the chemo.

My range of motion and strength are better, although not 100%, particularly after each saline fill for three to four days. The progress has allowed us to feel hopeful, but we are just trying to handle this one day at a time.

— Jenny

Hi! I walked in the 2009 LA Revlon Run/Walk today. I was very moved by the men and women who were there in memory of those who have died, or in honor of loved ones who are survivors, as well as by the thousands of courageous survivors who walked proudly with me. I wore a lanyard with your photo and Karen's photo. I shared it with whomever I spoke.

Happy Mother's Day! — Molly

There is one detail from the trip to New Hampshire that merits mentioning. Because each tissue expander had a large metal disk where saline was injected during the reconstruction, I was very concerned about airport security. The hidden metal could have turned security checkpoints into a nightmare. I traveled with documentation, but I was still afraid I would need to undress in front of a shocked airport security employee. I was hoping the person in question would at least be a female. At that point my reconstruction was lumpy, asymmetrical, and rather abnormal. If a total stranger had seen it, the experience would have been humiliating. Gladly I did not have to face the dilemma.

∞

No Chemotherapy Needed! A Teen-Blog Entry

May 14th

BUENAS NOTICIAS (Spanish for good news)

Hola gente!!!! (Hello popleee!) Mi madre does not need chemo! You know what that means right??? SHE'S KEEPING HER HAIR yay :) (Don't lie. You were all worried). This means my father will remain the only bald one in the house!! woohoo :)))))) The result of her Oncotype DX test was a 5%! Ha ha she failed :) just kidding! For this test the lower the number the better. 100% is the worst! I wish it was like that in school :(

She started to exercise (whimpily if I might add), but she's still cool 'cause she has a credit card. I'm not cool. I still remain without one :(

*OH YEAH, for Mother's day she got these cool breast cancer
slippers, and she gave them to me :))) She also got a camera, which I
might take. Hehe ... Just kidding, I'm not THAT mean. But she's sooo
lucky her type of cancer has its own clothing line and a pretty color. It
would've been so boring if it were not a fashionable cancer. My father is
handsome ... he told me to put that.*

*Well joking aside, we're happy with the test results and with her
progress. We appreciate your good wishes and prayers :) but don't
forget to keep the food coming :) peace :) I hope you guys know who
wrote this. If not, you really shouldn't be reading this* ☺

An early-stage diagnosis, with either negative lymph nodes or with a few positive ones, along with an estrogen-receptor positive (ER+) status, is the Oncotype
DX eligibility criteria. A low Oncotype DX score meant I would derive little or no
benefit from chemotherapy. Before that diagnostic tool, chemotherapy would have
undoubtedly been recommended.

⤜⤛

LIFE IN THE MIDST OF RECONSTRUCTION

May 24th

*As posted by Nicole, I received the long-awaited Oncotype DX
results. Even though chemotherapy was ruled out, I still got very
emotional—some days inexplicably are. The emotional roller coaster is
part of this territory, though it still catches me by surprise. I am seeing
things from a different perspective. Even emotions like gratitude and
contentment can feel overwhelming.*

*Without saline fills my comfort level should increase. I still need
to sleep upright, although a memory wedge has eased the discomfort.
Surgery might help. The implants will be smaller, less rigid, and more
comfortable than the expanders. I've not forgotten about thank-you
notes, I know I have many to write. My handwriting is improving as my
pectoral discomfort lessens. When that happens, I will contact those of
you who have been so generous, and again, I am sorry for the delay.*

*We are regaining a semblance of normality. These days we are
feeling less stressed, projects around the house are once again getting*

noticed, and we are starting to socialize. Some evenings we have teenagers in our house until late. Our pool and Ping-Pong table are getting a workout, but they are not the only ones enjoying the pool. Sandy, Magic, and I are in it nearly every day. I am going to miss it when I have surgery. In a few weeks Nicole will be going on a cruise with a friend, and Neil will be attending an engineering camp. He will also be getting his license in a few days, which means we have been looking for cars. It is good to be doing research on something other than breast cancer!

I've been reflecting on how perfectly poised and balanced our young adults have been. They've been supportive, helpful, and caring. All while maintaining their sense of humor, friendships, time for themselves, and for us, as well as their high academic standards. What a joy they are, and how they have chosen such respectful, caring individuals as their friends. It is great to have the house full of teenagers again.

At their respective schools, we recently participated in the annual 'Relay For Life' events, which raised funds for the American Cancer Society. I had previously volunteered, attended, and chaperoned, but clearly, I had never attended as a survivor.

I am sensing pins and needles under my left arm and axilla, perhaps the prelude to sensation. In a few days I might feel safe enough to drive. Today my discomfort will increase yet again with another saline fill, but the last few days have felt miraculous. — Jenny

The Relay For Life events were my first public appearances as a breast cancer survivor. The experiences were emotionally and physically challenging, but the wish to emulate you—my new sisters, the multitude of breast cancer survivors—started to emerge. Your courage and passion for the breast cancer cause began to inspire me.

❧

THE BENEFITS OF MEDITATION AND VISUALIZATIONS

When the Oncotype DX anxiety passed, I started to operate under a foreign sense of joy from frequent meditations. I highly recommend meditation.

Meditation helped me to find emotional strength, allowed me to find joy, and provided pain reprieves. Once I relaxed by making sure my mind and body were in a soothing state, I would focus on relaxing specific painful areas with inhalation and on releasing the pain with exhalation.

It was not just meditation. Through specific visualizations I started to see my world in a different manner. I frequently visualized putting on glasses. The spectacles focused on present enjoyments, filtered out future fears, and they intermittently let sadness in to keep it real. I would close my eyes and command a more positive perspective as I reopened them, and I instructed each breath to help do the same. Much later, as I started to rehabilitate, I visualized strength returning to weaker muscles.

It is impossible to describe just how powerful those simple techniques really are. I could always ease my pain, and even though they were temporary, the reprieves stabilized my sanity. There was always humor, beauty or joy to be found, even on stressful days. Calmness can be cultivated under challenging circumstances.

⊗⊗⊚

LESSONS LEARNED FROM DIAGNOSTIC SCREENINGS

June 5th

Since a friend is about to embark on this same sad journey, the stress of this situation is suddenly undeniable. My heart aches for her—I've cried more for her than I did for myself. There is some consolation in knowing that my experience encouraged her to seek additional screenings, and that our medical connections will serve as a guide. Others have suggested I share what I've learned, so here it goes on this blog.

Mammograms are important, but if at all possible make sure yours are DIGITAL. With that technique the radiologist can zero in on areas of concern. Close to 20% of breast cancers are missed by mammograms, in part because not all of them calcify. If you bring previous films, the comparison makes it easier to detect changes.

If your mammogram is normal find out if there is DENSE tissue, it may not be included in the report. If you have a LOT of dense tissue, you or your doctor may want to pursue additional screenings.

A DIAGNOSTIC mammogram can provide some answers, although it involves more compression and views. An ULTRSOUND might be worth seeking if you have a lot of dense tissue—that's how my lesion was seen. If still in doubt, an MRI can help sort things out, and a BIOPSY can decide for sure.

Don't forget to follow your instincts, listen to your body, and know your breast tissue well. The combination is responsible for my timely diagnosis. Young women, especially those with any type of family history, should be vigilant. Even men should be watchful, particularly if there is breast cancer in their family. Over 1900 men are diagnosed with breast cancer every year in the United States. Early detection, starting with regular self-exams, is the key. In other words, be on your guard!

— Jenny

❦

IMPLANT DECISIONS: SILICONE VS. SALINE

Important reconstructive issues were absent from the blog. Since I had always avoided plastic surgery due to possible risks, the need to rely on implants made me angry; although, the sentiment only surfaced when I had to make the final decisions. To put my mind at ease from a recurrence perspective, I searched for long-term studies on those of us who reconstruct with implants while at an early stage. Luckily I found reassuring information [98].

The anxiety did not end there. I was concerned about the type of implant fill I should choose. I initially wanted saline implants, but my silicone concerns seemed unfounded. Silicone implant research was extensive. Gel-filled implants were considered safe enough to be approved by the FDA in 2006, for both cosmetic and for reconstructive purposes [25]. It also became clear that most implant replacements (on newly designed implants) were for size changes or as a result of capsular contractures [152]—not because of leaks or ruptures.

My plastic surgeon wisely steered me towards silicone. He asked me to find mastectomy patients satisfied with saline implants. I was unsuccessful, although from the attempt I understood that a previous neighbor had been unhappy with her cosmetic outcome after a double mastectomy, at least until she exchanged her saline implants for silicone. Much later I found information confirming that on average, mastectomy patients who reconstruct with implants are more satisfied with silicone than they are with saline [25,109].

※

SLOW PROGRESS

June 9th

I have to pace myself. Rushing sets me back for days, I've learned the hard way. Working out these days consists of stretches, light yoga, limited range of motion, and short walks. I need to focus on comfortable movements, test new limits gently and gradually, and massage tight muscles frequently. I will lose ground with surgery but I am determined—I will do whatever it takes to maximize my comfort. Although, perhaps because I still have such limited sensation to the back of my arms, axillae, or to portions of my back, movement above shoulder level is not possible. Lymph node removal might be responsible for the numbness. I have less sensation on the left side, the very axilla that lost six lymph nodes, and I have more sensation on the right one, which lost only four. I do not believe this is permanent. Since so much progress has taken place, continued improvement might be the natural progression.

The medical highlight of the week will be a consult with a medical oncologist. She would have been in charge of my chemotherapy, but since that has been ruled out we will be discussing anti-estrogen therapy. Even though I have concerns about the potential side effects, I am willing to listen to the experts and look at the statistics. I want to see if the numbers are convincing. Wish me luck!

Each day seems brand new, worrying about trivial things suddenly seems irrelevant. I will strive to maintain the gift of gratitude, one positive outcome from this challenging experience. Happy summer everybody!

— Jenny

※

No Anti-Estrogen Therapy!

June 18th

I was needlessly concerned. The meeting with the medical oncologist went better than anticipated. Aromatase inhibitors, or postmenopausal anti-estrogen therapy, would have blocked estrogen availability in my body for 5 years. Many people tolerate this important therapy well, but others are not as lucky. Those of us with a difficult premenopausal experience (and a history of the potential side effects) are more likely to experience undesirable symptoms.

Luckily I had a rare type of breast cancer. Assuming there is no lymph node involvement, it seldom spreads beyond breast tissue. In other words, I had a good type of cancer. It was hard to detect, but the prognosis is relatively good at an early stage.

I never thought the medical oncologist would agree that in my case, the risks could outweigh the benefits. The anti-estrogen therapy would only decrease my recurrence rate from 5% to 3%, not enough to risk so many health problems. It feels as though a big weight has been lifted off my shoulders. She recommended exercise, a good diet, and vitamins, go figure.

Having this off my mind will make Monday seem minor by comparison. It is a two-hour general anesthesia procedure. I should be home by noon or so, and then the finish line of this marathon might seem within my grasp. I will not come in first, nor unfortunately last, although I will always hold my participatory badge with pride.

Since this surgery is the last stage of my treatment, I am looking forward to it. Sandy will not be working that week, but with Neil driving, with the kids out of school, and with my recovery expected to be speedy, life should be back to normal soon. As I prepare for my hopefully short sabbatical, music, good books, my family's sense of humor, and the positive wishes from my large and wonderful village, have the capacity to make this last step a breeze. Thanks in advance!

— Jenny

Even though my Oncotype DX result was low, it was still unclear whether anti-estrogen therapy could be avoided. The tumor was larger than anticipated, the cancer had spread throughout several milk ducts, and one of my margins was close, although still acceptable.

Since the standard of care in most literature (for my cancer size and stage) was chemotherapy followed by an aromatase inhibitor, I did not think I would get away without receiving at least one of them. I strongly believed neither was necessary, although for a while, my instincts did not appear defensible.

I spent many hours researching. I considered personal and family history, type of cancer, possible side effects, surgery, and Oncotype DX results. My *family* history of uterine cancer, arthritis, osteoporosis, high cholesterol, depression, and heart disease, all pointed to increased side effects. The same was the case with my *personal* history of headaches, hot flashes, joint and muscular aches, although my recent menopause, and my promise to exercise frequently, also played a role in the decision.

I also learned that my specific type of breast cancer (*tubular*) might not require anti-estrogen therapy or chemotherapy; it seldom spreads beyond breast tissue if lymph nodes are negative for cancer, although the development of a second (more aggressive) primary breast cancer on the opposite breast has been noted [134]. A double mastectomy was a good decision in my situation. The tubular breast cancer was a mixed blessing. It was a slow grower, and it made anti-estrogen therapy avoidance less concerning, but since it was soft to the touch and it did not calcify, the diagnosis was challenging.

I was thrilled. Such a reputable medical oncologist considered my input. We agreed to do CT scans of the chest and abdomen in case they are ever needed for comparison. The outcome of that appointment left me feeling like I just won the lottery, when in reality all I gained was the ability to keep what little estrogen my menopausal body was still producing. And yet, that was all I was hoping to derive from the consultation. A different outcome could have had a negative impact on my quality of life for a number of years.

❧

A FINAL THANK YOU

June 24th

I want to do more than I probably should. My range of motion has increased, the chest tightness has improved, and even though it will take a while, full mobility might again be the norm.

It seems important to acknowledge how instrumental the blog has been, even though it has fulfilled its purpose. It not only kept all of you, our dear friends and family members informed; it encouraged me to find positive angles at every turn so they could be reported in that manner, which was very therapeutic.

Breast cancer is now part of my life. Follow-ups will take place, and I will need to confront plastic surgery incidentals. Through it all I will try to enjoy this wonderful life that I've been granted, along with its many blessings. I've learned more than medical lingo. I've become well acquainted with the power of kindness, and with the responsibility of paying it forward with the same currency.

Since those definitions are so personal and individual, I have not elaborated on the spiritual aspects of my experience; nonetheless, I would like to urge all of you to stay open to that guidance, particularly in your hours of need. Don't ever forget about the power of your caring, your prayers, and your good wishes. They've not only contributed to my mental, spiritual, and to my physical sense of well-being, they've supported my family. You have taught our children the true meaning of the word "community." Indeed, the best things in life are not things at all ... Thank you!

Part Three

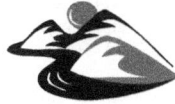

Introspection

(Or internal perception) is the detailed mental examination of one's conscious thoughts and feelings.

(Wikipedia)

THE JOURNAL:
ADDITIONAL SURGERY, COMPLICATIONS,
AND ATYPICAL RESOLUTIONS
June 2009-March 2011

"We can never obtain peace in the outer world until we make peace with ourselves"
— The Dalai Lama

"Peace comes from within. Do not seek it without."
— Buddha

Repressed anger and frustration have many faces and none of them are pretty. I had been trying to bottle up my negative emotions, but that option no longer sufficed. I knew I needed more surgery when I closed the blog, I just could not share the setback.

I was still lucky. Blogging led to journaling when I needed an outlet. You too might want to consider journaling. A purposeful activity felt like a lifeline in the midst of so many difficult emotions. I didn't know it then, but journaling helped me to cope with the stress of additional surgery, prolonged pain, emotional upheavals, and spiritual bewilderment. My journal became a good place to vent unwelcome cancer suspicions. I documented mobility challenges and muscular imbalances. Writing allowed me to organize my medical information, which in time led to this project. Many months passed in that fashion, including my first anniversary as a breast cancer survivor. At that point my journal was a collection of reconstructive information, personal feelings, and rehabilitative efforts. The journal continued to evolve—my healing was not complete. By the end of my second survivorship year I started to overcome many of my seemingly insurmountable obstacles, through a great deal of introspection, research, complementary approaches, and unwavering perseverance. It also happened because for the first time in my life, I became well acquainted with my inner warrior.

A note to the reader: To enhance accuracy, limit repetition, and enhance comprehension, it was necessary to edit and in some instances merge initial journal entries.

~

THE NEED TO JOURNAL

June 28th 2009

I need to retreat. I need privacy to grieve my latest setback. I know why I did not want to share my disappointment on the blog. I've never felt comfortable being on the receiving end of any equation, not even for the past few months. From the time of my diagnosis I have been trying to protect others by making light of things, by keeping a strong front, and by going out of my way to reassure everyone. And even though that is still a part of who I am, right now I lack the energy to protect anyone else. I have nothing left to give.

I wrongly assumed I was done with surgical procedures for a while, but that will not be the case. I am asymmetrical and I have a capsular contracture. I also developed a *hematoma*, and the bleeding under the skin created another layer of asymmetry. Since the unevenness is noticeable through clothing, and the idea of waiting six more weeks seems unbearable, I wanted my plastic surgeon to perform the revision within days. He wisely declined. Two surgeries in such a short period would increase my chances of an infection, although he still had to deal with my disappointment. Reconstructive surgery must demand a lot of patience.

Needing assistance for this long has felt odd, unfamiliar, and even uncomfortable at times. I need to rethink my dependency issues, though that will be hard and will take time. My needs will have to remain a priority for a while, but that too seems depressing. Maybe I can start by realizing that I am not always able to control or predict situations—another scary concept.

I am not ready to verbalize these feelings. Instead, I will explore my thoughts in this personal journal. I am hoping journaling will be as cathartic as I have always heard it can be. If it is, I might regain my focus. Journaling might prove to be all of those things. I found the introspection necessary to write the blog entries healing, and even though sitting and typing are uncomfortable positions, the impulse to document my feelings is much, much stronger than avoiding the pain. Cancer still has things to teach me, although I am also sensing those lessons won't be easy ones to learn.

MEDICAL MANAGEMENT DISAGREEMENT

June 30th

As difficult as it was to arrive at the conclusion, Sandy can no longer participate in my medical decisions, or go to doctors' appointments with me. Why didn't I notice we had such opposite views? In retrospect there were clues. At one point he questioned my research without offering assistance. When he realized that I will be questioning what could have been done differently, our difference of opinion reached a new level.

Once I removed my emotions I understood. In his view a good patient should find a good doctor, listen to the advice, and follow instructions without controversial comments. That's his style. Not just because of what he was taught in medical school from the doctor's perspective, it's his approach at his own medical appointments. I can understand that from a professional angle, but not from a personal one. I cannot be that type of patient. I *have* to be involved. Not just because there are so many options to choose from, but because all of them are so consequential. My questioning is not intended to be disrespectful—I'm only interested in joint dialogue.

There might be another explanation. This was the first time we got angry at my diagnosis and at how it has disrupted our lives, although we did not need to get angry at each other. We usually give in to the partner who feels the strongest about a subject, but since we both have strong opinions, we are on plan B: agree to disagree. This situation reminds me of one in Geralyn Luca's *Why I Wore Lipstick to My Mastectomy.* She describes how her husband (also a physician) had trouble coping with the medical aspects of her breast cancer treatment. For a time, she had to accept his withdrawal and attend appointments without him [106]. Evidently there is more to this than meets the eye.

⁂

CANCER'S EFFECT ON 20TH WEDDING ANNIVERSARY

July 4th

Yesterday was our 20th anniversary, but thanks to breast cancer the day was very different from what we once hoped—we wanted to be on a romantic trip to Spain. My recent surgery narrowed the celebratory options, and a trip was out of the question. Still, it seemed important to recognize 20 years of marriage in some upbeat fashion, even though I was exhausted and we were still at odds with each other. As a compromise of sorts we opted to go away for the night, except even that became challenging from a physical perspective.

Those were not the only things threatening to make our 20th anniversary a greater challenge than it should have been. I have of course been feeling uncomfortable about the way I look as a result of the asymmetry, the capsular contracture, the hematoma, and from the impossible to ignore incisions. Though there was still another barrier; after the reconstructive surgery I saw a look in Sandy's eyes that resembled disappointment. I cannot blame him if he is disappointed, I am.

Luckily this sad story has a happy ending. When we were enjoying an amazing meal at our favorite restaurant, we realized that by anyone's definition we've had a great marriage and a couple of unbelievable kids. Despite our recent health upheavals, we have been lucky. The sense of gratitude allowed us to reconnect. Our anniversary will still be remembered in a positive light, even without our dream getaway.

Our short getaway gave us a brief break from our breast cancer stress and we remembered what matters most: even though we have different opinions, and we are experiencing a breast cancer disruption, our love for each other (and for our children) remains our true constant. Our anniversary has empowered us. We will not let breast cancer destroy what we have built together for over 20 years.

❧

INCREASED DISCOMFORT & LACK OF PROGRESS

July 23rd

Day-to-day difficulties are increasing, rather than diminishing. The discomfort is more intense than before the last surgery, though this time there is an added bonus: my upper arms hurt a lot, particularly the back of my left upper arm. More disruptive is the fact that I have almost no strength in either arm, particularly my left one. It looks like skin on bone. Some muscles in that arm do not even contract when I try to flex them. Wearing a seatbelt has become impossible and driving is very difficult. The left-sided weakness is especially challenging; before breast cancer I was left-handed, a habit that is proving hard to break.

I cannot exercise frequently—that would be extremely tiring. I can no longer run. Running increases the torso tightness, although I knew my running days would eventually end. I can walk short distances, though very slowly. Muscle tightness prevents reaching behind my head. I frequently stretch and reach beyond my comfort level, but the tension still recurs. As expected, without the aggressive stretches I used to perform, my upper back is not accepting my present limitations gracefully.

Understanding the cause of so much discomfort would help, but the reason is not clear. Nerve trauma from the loss of six lymph nodes on the left side could be contributing, and the tightness on the right side might be from the capsular contracture. My limited shoulder motion is definitely adding pain, and the combination might be slowing lymphatic drainage. To limit muscular tension, improve shoulder motion, and lessen scar tissue, I frequently massage tight muscles and perform frequent range of motion exercises. To help lymphatic drainage I constantly elevate my arms and massage them towards my torso. I am also avoiding tight shirts.

In light of the next surgery progress seems pointless, though if I stop I might develop more scar tissue, get even weaker, and face a longer recovery. The added surgery will not help, but it is also clear that we all progress at different paces. I have to remain patient and stay focused on the ultimate goal.

At home I can reach important items and everyone helps so I don't have to overstrain, but away from that comfort zone I felt handicapped. Last week we spent six days in New Jersey with family. And even though I enjoyed seeing everyone, particularly my beloved mother-in-law Edith, sitting for hours at a time made me feel like I was in a torture chamber. In a fixed position the pain radiates to my back and neck. Not being able to hold the newest baby in the family was sadder than sad. My inability to tour schools in New York City with Sandy and Neil because I felt so tired was humbling and depressing. There was one small silver lining. When I tried to wear sleeves, I realized my pain increases with fitted sleeves, even if they are only worn briefly.

This roller coaster has made the cliché "how are you doing?" difficult to answer. I no longer provide an explanation. I have settled for the less complicated "fine" as a response, which is the best reply. I've worn out my sympathy card with most people. That's unfortunate; I will again need to rely on others, even though the concept seems embarrassing and imposing.

I am in uncertain territory. Even though everyone believes I am progressing well, so many day-to-day difficulties and fatigue do not seem normal. It does not feel like I am progressing, not at all.

Asymmetry

July 25th-27th

For the appearance of symmetry an insert is necessary on the right side. Due to the lack of sensation I was afraid to use pins, but then the insert would shift without my knowledge. I finally sewed an insert into a couple of bras. That helped, although I am still feeling self-conscious, even with loose shirts. The asymmetry is particularly apparent with the many slightly fitted T-shirts I own, although due to the renewed discomfort, I am again wearing my large post-mastectomy shirts.

Reconstructive asymmetry is *not* preventable. My suspicion was confirmed by an engineering college brochure intended for Neil. The pamphlet describes how one student is trying to design a device that can reduce the need for "visual" decisions, lower revision surgeries, and take "three-dimensional measurements" before mastectomies [172]. Three-dimensional measurements would also be useful for post-operative asymmetries such as mine. There is some consolation in knowing that I am not alone with this troublesome issue, which most people would not want to discuss.

Mastectomy patients develop more capsular contractures than patients who receive implants for strictly cosmetic reasons. We form more scar tissue when our skin is forced to attach to our pectoral muscles. My plastic surgeon explained that many capsular contractures resolve with aggressive massages. I've not been in that lucky majority.

I finally understand why, aside from the capsular contracture, I was disappointed with my cosmetic result. During the reconstruction the outcome could still improve, but when the permanent implants were in place, that was no longer the case. I was also not prepared for how different the round implants would look, as opposed to the teardrop expanders. All of that explains why my body image issues surfaced after my reconstructive surgery, and just when I thought they would be fading.

It seems as though with tissue expanders, the opportunity to develop asymmetry remains throughout the entire process. Saline travels via the path of least resistance with every fill, just like any other fluid would. The process (intended to stretch skin and pectoral muscles) is more likely to happen unevenly if either scar tissue or swelling develop. According to my tissue report, the weight of the tissue removed from each side resembles the asymmetry. Although, my plastic surgeon explained that many of us are not symmetrical prior to our mastectomies. In other words, the surgery is not necessarily incomplete. This theory has provided an explanation, and since there isn't a scientific method to determine the size of the implants, I am going to let it play a role.

A revision is the right choice for me. I am glad to finally feel so certain; I was concerned about the inconvenience for everyone involved. The prospect of having to recuperate from yet another surgery is not appealing, but staying this unhappy with how I look dressed and undressed is not acceptable. I want to make peace with my body.

✑

Metastatic Cancer Fear

July 29th

The scans from July 24th left me in a stressful limbo. The chest scan was clear, which is great, considering that my lungs are in proximity to the close cancer margin. On the other hand, the abdominal scan revealed several liver spots.

Part of the anxiety can be blamed on the impending surgery, the anticipated setbacks, and on the possible complications. On some days I am able to stay positive, but most of the time my fears still manage to surface, no matter how hard I try to keep them at bay. I am still glad for my early stage diagnosis, for not needing chemotherapy, radiation, or hormone suppression, but for some reason, none of those usually comforting details are helping.

I am not willing to share such potentially concerning news with most people, including our children. Sandy and I agreed; we should not ruin the rest of their summer without knowing for sure. My wish to keep the liver scan report private reminds me of when I discontinued the blog, except this time I contacted a couple of friends. My friend Tatiana has been a good listening board, even though her double mastectomy was just 10 days ago. We are at different stages in our recovery, but we still understand each other in ways our husbands cannot. Gilda Radner was right, "it's always something," although right now, there are way too many things happening at once.

✑

Informed Implant Decisions

August 1st-4th

Over six months ago I searched for nipple-sparing mastectomy visuals, and although I found a few photos, detailed information was limited and that has not changed. Most internet searches for implant sizing still produce visuals of cosmetic augmentations, even though I specifically typed the word *mastectomy*. Such findings have been frustrating and pointless. Implants look completely different on women with breast tissue. The weight of the patient, the implant shape, and even the size of the implant are usually not listed, even though each changes the outcome.

This time I feel prepared to make most of the implant decisions. I can now focus only on this one issue, I have a better understanding of the choices, and I know my body better than anyone. Luckily my plastic surgeon feels comfortable with my involvement. Since the ultimate goal is to create a natural look for someone my age and size, I am taking into consideration the asymmetry, the achieved expansion, my previous bust contour, the width of my torso, the size of the implants, and where my natural breast crease lies. The time between the surgeries has obviously been good. The swelling and the bleeding subsided, and that gave us a better sense of the asymmetry. I looked for information on the product website, and to make sure the implant diameter is a good fit for my small chest cavity, I've done a lot of measuring. I put together a final chart, which my plastic surgeon seemed to enjoy.

We kept two previous choices: the silicone fill, because it does feel very natural, and the round shape without texture. Even though the profile is enticing, we again ruled out the *contoured-teardrop* implants. If those implants rotate, surgery is necessary to reposition them [151]. Not an appealing prospect at this or at any other time.

Once I settled on the shape and the fill, I had to choose the projection. I had to consider that the *low*-profile implants are flatter and wider in diameter, not unlike I used to look. But the wide base might prove too large for me and could reach the nerve-sensitive areas below my left axilla. Besides, my plastic surgeon does not like to use the low-profile ones often; he explained that some projection is lost during the first year. The next choice was the high-profile implant, though I quickly discarded that possibility. Their high projection would look unnatural in someone my age and size. Their base diameter is also the narrowest, and the spacing between them would create a foreign look. In the end I chose the *moderate-projection round-silicone* implants. I am hoping their medium base diameter, along with their moderate projection, will be my best option.

The only thing I can do now is hope for a good cosmetic outcome, without complications. I will redirect my focus. I will prepare my body, our family, and our house for my third round of limitations.

MASTECTOMY SCARS & FEMININITY

August 11th

To get in the right frame of mind for my next sabbatical, and hoping to take advantage of the last few days of summer, last week we traveled to the north end of South Beach. Unlike the south portion, that area has access to the boardwalk and less topless women. I was planning on having location-appropriate conversations with our nearly grown teenagers, the very ones that might have been avoided in a different setting.

I had always tried to teach our children that *physical appearance should not determine self-esteem.* I modeled a healthy body image by exercising, by eating well, by avoiding conversations that revolved around physical characteristics, and with plastic surgery avoidance. Then thanks to breast cancer I sought plastic surgery. I now have two five-inch scars in case I ever want to forget why they are there.

I had never considered going topless, but last week I entertained the possibility. I wanted to make the statement that I am just as feminine as every other woman is, even though I now have mastectomy scars. We, the mastectomy patients, should not be ashamed of having scars, any more than anyone else is of other types of scars. No, I did not do it, and not because of my reconstruction; my husband and children deserve some respect. My scars might have been well received in South Beach—the atmosphere is of acceptance.

The trip was a good decision. Spending time with my middle brother and sister, whom I hardly ever get to see, was enjoyable and distracting. The sun, the gorgeous beaches, and the walking felt healing and empowering. The entire experience put me in a positive frame of mind for the surgery. I am finally excited about the potential outcome.

෧෪෨

DEFIANT ATTITUDE AFTER THIRD SURGERY

August 15th

My amazing cosmetic outcome was worth the wait!

The surgery was a success. I had no bleeding or any other complications. The incisions, which have been cut three times, look better than anticipated, probably because the cutting was done along the exact same lines. I am tired and nearly pain free, and yet I know the drill from last time: the pain will reemerge when I need to drive, cook, and be active. I tried to be more realistic. I was hoping to prevent another disappointment, although even without that preparation, I would not have been disappointed. I look more symmetrical. I feel more *normal*.

Even though it will be challenging, I will refrain from lifting and driving, as is recommended. Besides, we are now experts. Yes, my limitations have become routine, although my family members are not mind readers. I have let them know when and how I need help. Expecting them to simply volunteer without asking is frustrating and unrealistic. That will be easier said than done, I tend to do everything myself, but again, I have no choice. I started by asking Neil if he would drive me to surgery. I wanted him to participate, and continue participating for the next six weeks, by performing the one adult privilege I just lost and he recently obtained—driving.

Before surgery I did all of the things that have now become routine, including getting a pedicure and a manicure. I picked the same bright neon pink color every time—my *FBC* color. In my manicure vocabulary that stands for f*** breast cancer. I wore that empowering nail polish to every important appointment, including my CT scan in July, and I plan on wearing it in a few weeks when I have the next scan. I also wore lipstick to all of my surgeries and got a great haircut, but that was not all. For reasons a therapist would enjoy analyzing, I wore beautiful lingerie to every surgery and I carefully applied my makeup. Those rituals reminded me I am still feminine, even though my body was being cut or scanned. The nail polish continues to work its magic two days after the surgery. It makes me feel defiant and determined, the very attitude I need as I try to progress.

⚬⚬⚬

Parenting Goals after a Friend Dies from Breast Cancer

August 19th

What feels like a breast cancer epidemic is touching many lives in our vicinity. On the day I was having surgery last week, Nicole was at a funeral for her friend's mother. The girls have known each other for a while, but their friendship truly strengthened as a result of their mothers' breast cancer. Apparently when Katie left her summer camp prematurely because her mother was dying, all of the girls wore pink for the rest of the day. The image easily formed in my mind. I have known many of the girls for over 14 years. The visual brought, and still brings, tears to my eyes.

Three weeks before she lost her struggle with breast cancer, I spoke with Katie's mom. I asked Nancy what she would have changed, as far as her kids were concerned, if she had the opportunity. She replied that she would have been more honest with them from the beginning. She wondered if a better understanding of her late-stage diagnosis would have made their acceptance easier towards the end, although without a doubt, her greatest regret was her inability to finish raising Katie. Nancy was very aggressive with her treatment, but her family believes dense tissue caused a late-stage diagnosis.

From her comment, I realized that at times I avoid in-depth conversations with our children. I often assume they are coping well if they look composed, even though that is not always the case. Teenagers tend to cope with their fears by denying them, and that can lead them towards troublesome behavior. I know why I've acted that way, especially if I am upset about a medical issue; as selfish as it sounds, it is easier to avoid those discussions. The avoidance doesn't always work. My body language, my tone of voice, and my topics of conversation give me away. Besides, our children are very intuitive, they seem to know when something is wrong. When I do speak clearly the honesty not only clears up the air; it also reinforces what I've tried to teach them: *when in doubt as to what to say, try the truth.*

I will try to improve my communication skills. I want our teenagers to learn that life's roller coasters are always easier when shared. During trying situations they are more likely to learn from me than they do at any other time. That's when they need my guidance the most. I will try to put some of my needs aside, become aware of theirs, and parent them properly.

Nancy did not get to finish raising her three kids. She was unable to accomplish that aim, the ultimate goal of every mother, everywhere. She sent two of her children to college, but not her third. Nancy was a wonderful woman, a loving wife, and a good friend to many. And yet, she will not get to see her youngest daughter start her sophomore year of high school, as I will get to do in a week. That's unfair. Nicole had to attend Nancy's funeral without either parent. That also seemed wrong, especially since I wanted to be there.

Nicole handled the experience as well as could be expected, in part because she is so vocal and expressive, although I also realized that she needs an occasional reminder: no one is exempt from a cancer recurrence, not even those of us with low recurrence percentages, regardless of how much she wants that to be the case.

Nancy my heart aches for you, for your family, and for your young Katie. This is unfair. In your honor I will try to improve my parenting skills, even though I am still facing obstacles. Your loss and your family's loss have served as reminders. The greatest joys are found in the simplest of moments, although I am so sorry I had to be reminded in this manner. You will be missed by many.

⨎

OUTPATIENT SURGERY TRENDS & MASTECTOMIES

September 5th

Before outpatient surgeries became the norm, most surgeries and breast reconstructions were performed in hospitals where patients spent several days recuperating. Aside from the obvious financial benefit, a decrease in surgery infections was one positive outcome.

But some things have been lost in translation, specifically nursing care and discharge instructions. When I was a registered nurse in the early 1980s, our discharge instructions took into account physical limitations. Patients who went home without assistance had to move around safely before being discharged; otherwise, we would contact social services to arrange at-home physical therapy, and/or visiting nurses. We expected basic food tolerance before discharge, and as a rule, we explained dietary restrictions. Medication interaction and narcotic weaning schedules were part of the package, as were alternate suggestions to help manage pain. Dressing and wound care were considered very important—patients or family members had to show us they could handle both before discharge.

That is not all. There is an even greater loss. Patients were able to ask surgical nurses questions about their recovery at a different time than right after surgery. That is now the norm in most outpatient facilities, while patients are still groggy from anesthesia and in pain. One possible solution would be to bring back the once mandatory class before surgery. For both of my reconstructive surgeries I was at an outpatient clinic. They did a great job with my anesthesia and my recovery, and for that I am grateful, but their discharge instructions were minimal at worst and standardized at best. That left me with essentially no information after one of the surgeries, when I was mistakenly given instructions for some type of nose procedure.

Tatiana and I were lucky to have an overnight stay for our double mastectomies. Yes, I said lucky. An insurance trend gaining national ground is encouraging same-day mastectomy discharges. Neither Tatiana, nor I, can envision our first night at home, and neither can our husbands. It was scary, painful, and confusing.

Sandy and I were surprised to encounter so many difficulties, particularly in a hospital setting.

Standard instructions are necessary. Nurses, just like every other health care professional, have become specialized. Health care costs need to be contained and in-hospital infection rates need to be reduced. Even so, I am hoping overnight stays will remain a possibility for those of us interested in that fading luxury. Hospitalizations provided the opportunity to discuss conflicting emotions with professionals trained in that difficult task.

⊸⊷

CANCER CHANGES PARENTING STYLE

September 10th

I am becoming the type of parent I always wanted to be—I am not as strict. It's not that I no longer discipline our children, I do. I even enforced limits when it seemed to add more stress after my diagnosis, as they still need boundaries and a sense of continuity. I am just picking my battles better and enjoying them more.

The new approach unexpectedly enhanced our communication and encouraged mutual honesty. On most occasions our teenagers are reasonable and responsible, but they mostly act that way after I treat them with respect and truly listen to their perspective. Nicole said I have "chilled." She explained that some of her friends want me to talk to their parents so they will do the same. Maybe she is right. A brush with death reminded me that parenting them is a privilege.

These days, I view my parenting role very differently. Rather than acting as their activity police officer, I want to help them learn from their mistakes. I tend to underestimate their judgment, although when given the opportunity, they usually rise to the occasion. They know I expect them to use their freedom wisely and that it is not guaranteed. They could lose ground if they make poor choices. Cancer is responsible for their newfound freedom and their sudden maturity. I don't have the energy to do everything for them or watch every move they make. By forcing them to become more responsible and involved, my challenges unexpectedly sped up their maturity.

I must be in denial about their impending adulthood. Last week I went through Neil's senior pictures. As his childhood flashed before my eyes, I found myself in tears. Helping him with college applications has also felt like a milestone—I am going to see him through his high school years. A few weeks ago we surprised

Nicole with a party for her 16th birthday. The realization that she and her friends look like such poised young ladies took me by surprise. She also has her first boyfriend. The relationship unexpectedly paved the way for various mother-daughter conversations, the very ones I expected later, although I am actually enjoying those discussions. I've not forgotten that some mothers do not live long enough to have them with their daughters.

Even if I never have a recurrence I will still not be in their lives on a daily basis, no matter how much they or I want that to be the case. The realization was initially upsetting, though in the end it prompted mutual appreciation. Their gratefulness may be short lived. I am not interested in ruining this period by being strict without a good reason.

Hopefully my new, improved parenting style is here to stay. It is not only more effective, it also *feels* right. The following poem by an anonymous author has been on my refrigerator for a number of years. It describes the kind of parent I always hoped to be, much better than I ever could.

If I had my child to raise all over again

I'd finger paint more and point the finger less.

I'd do less correcting and do more connecting.

I'd take my eyes off my watch and watch with my eyes.

I would care to know less and know to care more.

I'd take more hikes and fly more kites.

I'd stop playing serious and seriously play.

I'd run through more fields and gaze at more stars.

I'd do more hugging and do less tugging.

I would be firm less often and affirm much more.

I'd build self-esteem first and the house later.

I'd teach less about the love of power, and more about the power of love.

❦

ONSET OF INTENSE NERVE PAIN

September 15th

Just when I thought things were starting to improve, I've taken a huge step back. It feels as though the skin on the back of my left arm, just off my axilla, and to a lesser extent on my chest, is on fire. Both surgeons reassured me; they explained that my nerves are trying to regenerate. I've unsuccessfully tried a couple of nerve pain pharmaceuticals, over-the-counter ointments, and my old narcotics, though all were a waste of time.

Getting dressed is suddenly very difficult. If anything comes in contact with the areas in question, a very strong, immediate burning sensation results. My entire wardrobe is suddenly obsolete. I frequently shop for something bearable to wear, except the exercise is as exhausting as it is futile.

Trying to function socially is by far the greatest challenge. Those who are not in pain cannot understand how I feel, any more than I can explain to them how much pain I am experiencing. I try to keep a "well front." Everyone is getting tired of the situation and most people feel helpless because they cannot offer solutions, except I often lack the energy, the pain is so draining. I am finding the typical "but you look good" response very inappropriate. What is that supposed to mean? It sounds like it is okay to be in pain, as long as I look well to the outside world. I know. The comment is meant to comfort me, and no one knows what to say, but "I am sorry" would at least validate the situation. I knew this would be a lonely journey, I just never knew how lonely.

⚜

UTERINE CANCER CONCERN

September 17th

The anxiety bar has been raised. At a recent doctor's appointment I reported that I've been experiencing postmenopausal bleeding—a sign of uterine or cervical cancer. The disclosure led to a vaginal/pelvic ultrasound three days ago.

Functioning for the past few days has been a real struggle. The new cancer fear; my intense, burning pain; and the unanswered liver scan questions are a challenging combination. Frustration, panic, and pain are intermingled in everything I do. I can never escape them—they are present everywhere I go. I usually prioritize the things I worry about and disregard all others, but suddenly, this new development has moved ahead of the previous runner-up: the unwelcome, painful burning sensation.

The Jewish New Year heightened my already elevated sensitivities. Emotionally I was moved when I asked G-d to inscribe me in the book of life for the coming year, as is traditionally done on this High Holy Day. Symbolically the day also had an enhanced meaning. From a health perspective, I felt the need to mark the New Year as a new beginning. I might try doing the same on December 31st and even on the Chinese New Year, if it will make a difference.

When I explained the latest development my kids were very supportive, although not surprised. My body language gave me away long before my spoken words did. After the appointment Nicole tried to distract me with small talk, just like she has been doing for months when she senses I need diversion. Neil is quieter and more reserved, but his facial expressions, extra kisses, long hugs, and those eyes of his say all that his lips do not. Neil has taught me that not all of us communicate in the same manner. I am no longer worried. Our one-way exchange is keeping him informed. Talking to them at once helps him in particular. Her questions give me a sense of what he might need to hear.

All of this is particularly burdening for Sandy. He is my safe place when I need to cry and get mad, as I inevitably did after the appointment. I explained that I am tired of being cut, scanned, and of being in pain, though most of all I am tired of so much uncertainty. I was glad when he listened and did not downplay the situation. He did not try to come up with a solution, as he usually tries to do. He would like to ease my worrying and my pain. He can't. He feels powerless. I understand, I too wonder how much more we will need to endure.

Even though I did not think anything could feel more overwhelming, living in fearful uncertainty is far more draining than living in constant pain.

⚜

COPING WITH UNCERTAINTY

September 21st

It is just after sunrise on a cloudless Monday morning. I have no idea if this exceptional day will bring any news regarding my latest procedure, but it can still be a good day. I can start by allowing the beauty around me to work its magic. The birds are singing, and even the air seems to be warming my very soul. They are reminding me that I am still here. They seem to know I will continue searching for health.

I have the gift of this day. I can either spend it in gratitude or in fear. Today I will be lucky enough to kiss my children good night, just like I was lucky enough to kiss them goodbye. That is what I will hold on to regardless of what today brings. Yes, I am stronger than I think I am. As this day unfolds, I will try to remember what Sandy always says: *the outcome of any event cannot be changed by worrying.*

Without my family's sense of humor, my multiple challenges would seem unbearable. Sandy's jesting makes him well-known and liked by many, particularly children. I never cease to be amazed. Neil and Nicole have been good students, although that is not surprising. They have been learning from the master. I try to participate, except for me, humor is difficult under the best of circumstances, and if my mood is as somber as it has been for the last several days, it is basically absent. Sometimes I wonder if they joke to lighten a situation or in spite of it. Either way, I am grateful and impressed. I know how they would respond to that statement; I am overthinking things, as that tends to be my style. My overthinking should not be underestimated. It provides valuable material for them to continue the verbal give and take.

The extra walking, my family's sense of humor, and my additional meditations are finally exerting a positive influence. I wish I could convince Sandy of how therapeutic these quiet spaces can be to calm fears and worries. I cannot. His clinical mind remains closed to such intangible concepts.

⚯

GRATITUDE

September 23th

I received the anticipated ultrasound report at 1 p.m., the exact time I was going to surgery six months ago. Inside the feared envelope I found yet another paragraph with the ability to change my life. I anxiously read the radiologist's conclusion, while noticing the power of the letters "a" and "b," which were luckily missing in front of the *normal* conclusion. My sense of relief was overwhelming, but then I was overcome by sadness for what I've endured in the past six months.

Once that feeling passed a sense of gratitude remained. At least for today I will not have to make any new appointments. Regardless of how nice and competent they might happen to be, I do not need to meet yet another set of cancer specialists. Not having to worry about uterine cancer made me feel like I rejoined the living, even in the midst of my pain. Every errand and task performed for the rest of the day was an absolute pleasure. I felt privileged to be performing activities that usually feel more like nuisances than blessings. What a great feeling! It was such a pleasure to share some good news with my family. Not even a hurricane could have taken away my sunshine on this day, the sixth-month anniversary of my double mastectomy.

⚈⚈⚈

REASSURANCE FROM RESEARCH

October 3rd-5th

Research made me a little more certain about being cancer-free, than many of my fellow cancer patients appeared to be in the radiology waiting room last week. Most of us did not look like cancer patients at all. In fact, we could have been a crowd at a restaurant where age, gender, weight, race, and socioeconomic status are not an issue.

When I had the courage to type the words *liver cancer*, I learned that it can either be *metastatic* or *primary,* and both appear unlikely. Primary liver cancer starts in the liver, and usually in individuals with liver cirrhosis, alcoholism, or hepatitis. None applies. That left the possibility of metastatic spread to the liver, although that too is unlikely with my type of cancer. Uterine or cervical involvement is a possibility, which is why I was so worried last week. In other words, my liver spots are probably benign, and apparently those are common and not dangerous.

A couple of days ago an oncology nurse practitioner validated my research. She stated that it would *"unheard of"* for my type of cancer to spread to the liver first. It is amazing how a choice of words can make or break a patient. I knew the spread to the liver was unlikely at this point, but unheard of? Now, that was reassuring!

If I need more confirmation an MRI would be the way to go, but the referral would need to come from my surgical oncologist. It was explained that I will not be going back to that practice, unless recurrence concerns are feared. Wow! I never thought I would be glad to have my patient status terminated at a physician's office, but I am thrilled. Many others have left those same hallways with a very different type of finality. I will not be pursuing an MRI. I am ready to end the testing merry-go-round. Besides, I now understand how difficult it must be for others to contemplate further treatment at a juncture such as this one, while still in pain and without strength and stamina.

Screening for cancer without metastatic symptoms is controversial. Screenings can lead to unnecessary worrying, but in my situation they were still instrumental. The ability to read reports suggesting that my lungs are clear, that there are no masses on my kidneys, and that I have a normal uterus have helped to restore my shattered health image. On the other hand, one recommending that "several liver lesions require follow-up to exclude metastatic disease" could not be overlooked. I might still develop metastatic cancer in the future, or I could have microscopic cancer now—no screening could rule that out. What I have is time right now. My cancer was the slow-growing type.

Some people do not benefit from screenings and research. I have. In the end, both brought more peace of mind than concerns. Avoiding testing is not always the easy way out, although it can be for some. I've spoken with some survivors who did not undergo additional screenings. Surprisingly, their lack of knowledge left them more worried about the whys and what ifs, than I have been.

Knowing that my liver spots are probably not metastatic disease is reassuring, but I also know the next time I sit in that radiology waiting room, Lady Luck might not be on my side. It all sounds depressing, but it was actually empowering. A wave of gratitude and a sense of urgency for the gift of time that is still mine washed over me. The sudden appreciation brought a joyful spring to my step that must have been very evident to others, as I walked away from my (hopefully last) medical oncology appointment, and quite literally, walked back into my life.

⬯⬯

FROZEN SHOULDER

October 8th

Not even I, a nurse, a reader, and an exercise enthusiast, escaped from immobility complications. To put it differently, a couple of weeks ago I developed a *frozen shoulder* on my left and weakest side. The increased left arm and shoulder pain, along with the new mobility restrictions, prompted stretch modifications, and a request for a physical therapy consult. My frozen shoulder is probably the result of limited strength and ongoing pain over an extended period of time, although the surgeries, the nerve damage, and the muscular imbalances also contributed. After the double mastectomy I had limited mobility in both arms, possibly from frozen shoulders, but persistent movement improved my range of motion.

Things are a little more complicated now. Dealing with a frozen shoulder, *and* having nerve pain in the same area, has been an interesting balancing act.

Heat and many of the recommended movements used to treat a frozen shoulder dramatically worsened the nerve discomfort. Since figuring out which exercises work best has been such a painful process, I've had to limit the interventions. To compensate, I am performing the least uncomfortable movements frequently and consistently, while trying to increase my reach gradually.

I have been enlightened. Frozen shoulders are considered *common* among breast cancer patients [153]. Evidently many patients have limited shoulder motion years after treatment. Some survivors might be under the wrong impression; they might assume a frozen shoulder is simply part of the breast cancer territory, and that nothing can be attempted.

My muscles and nerves seem to have opposite needs. This is a balancing act that must be performed with care. If I cannot find a way to increase my mobility I might develop more scar tissue. Even though it is difficult, I have to persevere.

⚘

Nerve Healing Progression

October 11th-14th

I now realize that the *extent* of my nerve damage, and my combined muscular weaknesses, are atypical after sentinel lymph node biopsies, and that nerve pain is very difficult to understand and even more challenging to treat.

Why did this happen? Perhaps if I can understand that I might comprehend what is going on, and if I can do that, then I will know what to do. In retrospect, having a bilateral mastectomy and two reconstructive surgeries in four and a half months was more than my body could gracefully handle. All the surgeries involved cutting through my pectoral muscles, general anesthesia, and ace bandages for weeks. To break up the capsular contracture scar tissue had to be removed during my third surgery, and that probably caused more swelling and healing challenges.

Specific symptoms could have sealed the nerve damage speculation. The first clue was that oral narcotics did not help. The second could have been the lack of sensation beyond the anticipated chest numbness; the back of my upper arms, my left axilla, and select back muscles, just beyond that axilla were numb. The third clue could have been that I had such limited mobility and nearly no strength. When some feeling graced my upper arms my range of motion increased, and the left arm nerve pain could then be traced along nerve paths. That joy was short lived. It was soon replaced by a constant burning sensation to the areas that lacked sensation.

The progression gives me reason to believe I am moving in the right direction, even though sometimes I take two steps forward and one step backwards. I need to be patient. My nerves are trying to regenerate. My medical team is hopeful and that is reassuring. Nerve pain can be permanent.

My arms have felt extremely heavy and weak. I've had to support them with small pillows when I sit, when I cross my arms, and even when I stand for more than a few minutes at a time. If I lift one pound, sit for too long, or drive for more than 10 minutes at a time, my left arm and chest are in pain within an hour, and often for several days afterwards. I've been unable to slice through a slice of French bread, open a sliding glass door, hold a book on my lap, or open a bottle of water, although last week I had an uncomfortable breakthrough: I pumped gas for the first time in over six months. My physical therapist thinks nerve disruptions are keeping specific muscles form moving and making my left arm feel heavy, and that mild lymphedema might be contributing to the sense of heaviness.

In my opinion, the wish to avoid long-term complications should be another reason to undergo frequent breast cancer screenings. The likelihood of all complications, including nerve damage, increases when more lymph nodes need to be removed [103] or when several therapies are combined. Since I only had surgery, I might have a good chance of recovering.

To symbolize just how little strength I've had over the past few months, and how it is ever so gradually coming back, I would like to document a scenario. I always stopped at the coffee shop in the medical oncology building as I exited, but since the creamers were positioned on a high shelf I experienced difficulties. I raised both arms every time, except my strength was essentially non-existent on June 18th and on July 24th. I swallowed my pride and asked strangers for help. On September 25th I was finally able to press the creamer pump but I had to use both hands, and yet even that made me feel accomplished and independent. On October 2nd I rushed to the coffee shop with joyful anticipation and I was not disappointed. Even though it was only with the right, I performed the task with just one hand.

Nerve pain understanding might be in its infancy. My new symptoms fit the description of *allodynia*, but information seems limited. Describing this development will take a while; I will tackle it on another day when I have more time. For now, I would like to reiterate that the constant nerve pain remains an ongoing challenge. I am assuming that if wearing sleeves causes discomfort, then my body might heal better without them. Luckily we live in Florida—my options would be more limited if it was otherwise.

Breast cancer treatment and reconstruction are not for the weak at heart, although in a roundabout way mine is getting stronger. I am more resilient than I ever believed I was.

❧

EMOTIONAL HEALING FROM A HOME PROJECT

October 16th

Sandy had last week off, and even though we need a vacation, we stayed home. Traveling is very challenging, I am very tired, and I need to stretch throughout the day. Part of me feels guilty for imposing limitations on my family, but the options feel limited.

We settled on a home project. Sandy needed a situation that he could control, that had a limited duration, and that offered clear results. He usually prefers to be in control and *fix* things. A sense of control is the opposite of what he has been experiencing through my surgeries, cancer scares, and lingering issues, all difficult experiences for any man to have to go through. Keeping in mind the possible benefits, and considering that woodworking is his favorite hobby, I agreed to let Sandy paint our room and upgrade the crown and floor molding. It would only be fair to mention that I was not happy with the idea of moving out of my comfort zone for the week, but now that the project is complete, I am elated with the results.

From the moment we stepped into the paint store it became clear that the project would also be therapeutic for me. Home improvement projects are the norm for people who are not dealing with cancer-related issues. At least for now, my definition of *normal* is anything unrelated to cancer screenings, research, treatment, reconstruction, pain management, and rehabilitation. I also felt normal because I looked normal. No one could tell I underwent a bilateral mastectomy a few months ago. I was probably seen as just a person with a home project. Perhaps my reconstruction has been worth the hassle.

The undertaking was good for our self-esteem, even though my contribution was limited. Other than ideas I was of little help, although I did update our window treatments with a colorful trim. Though quite painful, sewing gave me a glimpse of my old self. Now that we are back in our room and our old pictures are in their new locations, the space feels new. It feels like a well room. It is amazing what a few wood strips and a fresh coat of paint can do. Both rejuvenated my sick space and gave us something concrete to do towards our much-needed emotional healing.

FIRST UNPRODUCTIVE PHYSICAL THERAPY ATTEMPT

October 18th-19th

I am feeling lost. Most recommendations, in either physical therapy or in breast cancer mobility literature, are not intended for nerve-related difficulties.

Soreness is expected when tight muscles and tendons are forced to stretch. I know. I've been experiencing that for months. It just seems that the discomfort should either be mild or provide some relief. Increased *severe* pain, the type that lasts for days at a time, seems altogether wrong. I tried to perform the strengthening exercises without bands or weights, though even then, the problem persisted.

My goal is simple. I want to function. That was downright impossible with the added layer of discomfort. I was forced to stop the therapy. The therapist was missing something about my situation. When I described the situation she had little else to offer, even though she is a lymphedema/mastectomy specialist.

Trying one motion at a time seems more beneficial. Isolating a movement lets me know if the pain improves, stays the same, or increases only temporarily. If any of those is the case I add it to my routine. I then repeat that cycle with yet another stretch, while starting with only a few repetitions at a time. To stay consistent I've been documenting the frequency of the movements and the angles as I am able to widen them. After a few days of that step-by-step process I have a limited number of exercises that are at least not setting me back and I do them religiously. I can only tolerate arm mobility for a couple of minutes at a time. My endurance barrier could have been part of the problem with the hour-long physical therapy sessions. I will reattempt weights and bands when some of my nerve pain diminishes. For now, I will focus on weightless range of motion in short intervals. This is humbling. I used to do so much more. My surgeons explained that it took months to lose the strength—that my nerve regeneration might still take a while—and that regaining lost strength might take even longer. I need to be patient.

⟡

ALLODYNIA (INTENSE BURNING NERVE PAIN)

October 21st-25th

It is time to elaborate on the term that I mentioned a few days ago. The discomfort on the back of my arms and on my chest fits the description: *Allodynia.* The term is a bit obscure. Even my smart computer is not recognizing it as part of the English language.

From what I've been able to gather, allodynia is an abnormal nerve response. It can make non-painful sensations, such as wearing clothes or a gentle touch, very uncomfortable [17]. It is not hypersensitivity. In that scenario, a typically painful sensation is even more painful. Allodynia can happen from chronic conditions, chemotherapy, metastasis, surgery, or when improper nerve healing takes place. According to my plastic surgeon even women who undergo breast augmentations can experience allodynia. It happens infrequently, but to insert the implants, nerves must also be cut. My allodynia feels like an intense burning sensation. It is aggravated by every type of contact, even soft fabrics. The allodynia is most noticeable in the back of my left axilla, where that arm attaches to my torso.

Even though they have side effects, anticonvulsants, antipsychotics, or antidepressants can help [126]. Limited relief, along with an extreme sense of sedation forced me to discontinue the ones I tried. They are also metabolized through the liver, which is concerning. There is another option: nerve blocks or trigger point injections. I will explore the possible benefits and side effects of both when I get a good pain specialist referral.

For now, my instincts are telling me to attempt the least-invasive methods. Covered ice packs to the most painful areas seem to help for short periods of time, although I have to be careful; my limited sensation might cause an ice burn. Dabbing rather than rubbing under my arms after a shower, and keeping hot water from touching the sensitive areas, seems worth the hassle. Shaving has become easier now that I found a small razor with a movable head, and a small roll-on deodorant is gentler than my old solid. The avoidance of fabrics near the affected areas has helped, although not nearly as much as frequent meditations and relaxation techniques.

I am afraid to get to know someone with permanent nerve pain in a support group. I've yet to find a success story for this level of nerve pain. I know healing potentials vary, but just reading similar, unresolved stories is very scary. My outcome could be different. Women treated before Oncotype DX technology (for the same cancer stage) might have undergone more therapies, which increases the likelihood of long-term pain.

Nerves have the capacity to slowly regenerate. My comfort level might improve, although the process could take up to two years. I've not ruled out aggressive methods. Those will be needed if conservative ones don't work. Deciding between further research, listening to my inner wisdom, and acting on any given choice feels like an intricate dance I must dance, whether I am in the mood to dance it or not.

CANCER BIRTHDAY SENTIMENTS

November 3rd

I am unusually excited. Today I look forward to celebrating the momentous occasion of my birth, on this, the 49th anniversary. My mood is atypical. I thought I was too old for birthday celebrations, but then came breast cancer. For the first time, in a long time, I am grateful for the miracle of aging. From this point forward, and for as long as I am blessed to celebrate this symbolic passage of time, I vow to honor it by spending it in gratitude. No, there will not be a party and I don't expect a deluge of phone calls. The order of business is lunch with my mother, a pedicure, and a quiet dinner with my family. The day will not be extraordinary, but it will be laced with an unusual sense of joy; I will celebrate myself.

Yes, I know. I am one year away from the dreaded half-century mark. That feared time when wrinkles and gray hair move to the top of most women's priority list. Even so, the idea of turning 50 is no longer concerning. Cancer was kind enough to show me the flip side of that coin. I now hope to someday look in the mirror and find a far more wrinkled version of myself, with nothing but beautiful white hair.

To age gracefully, I used to search for role models in older women. Not anymore. These days I admire all of my older female counterparts. I wish it was socially acceptable for me to tell them how beautiful they are, even with their unique imperfections. We are a society obsessed with perfect bodies, but now when I see women with imperfect curves, I see their true beauty: those bodies are their own. Reaching maturity with an intact body is a health attribute that should be celebrated. Perfection should not be the only goal. Imperfect is how we are supposed to look in the second half of our lives, after our bodies have completed their intended reproductive tasks, and we give ourselves back to ourselves.

Aging is a privilege. In time I hope to be part of that elite group. I dream of seeing our kids graduate from high school *and* from college. I want to dance at their weddings. I would love to watch Andrew make the environmental footprint he hopes to make, and I want to see Neil become the amazing man he is meant to become. I would like to be there when all of their babies are born, and even though it sounds sexist, I dream of counseling Nicole. I want to help her when she struggles to cope with the challenges of a newborn and with the trials of breast feeding. I want to buy birthday presents for my future grandchildren and read to them until they fall asleep on my lap. I even dare to envision Sandy and me in our golden years, with enough strength to babysit our grandchildren, and with enough health to travel together.

Other cancer survivors feel birthdays have been rediscovered. Just last week I saw an older African-American woman in a magazine wearing a birthday crown. She was beaming. She could have lit up the sun. That radiant face probably stirred similar sentiments in other cancer survivors. She represents the American Cancer Society's *More Birthdays Campaign*, a fundraising effort with a very appropriate website: morebirthdays.com.

❧

IMPLANT MIGRATION

November 5th-7th

It seems as though my once-strong pectoral muscles have lost most of their muscle tone and have been nearly dormant. The weakness has been an inconvenience, but then it became a much bigger problem in late September. My right pectoral muscle and the surrounding skin overstretched, causing the right implant to migrate below the incision line by approximately two inches. My hard-earned symmetry was distorted. Reaching above my head worsened the problem, and that presented a difficult dilemma; I needed to stretch. I struck a compromise by bending forward, which seems to disengage the pectoral muscles.

My plastic surgeon explained that it usually takes two to three weeks of binding for the implants to settle and for the pectoral muscles to heal. Prior to me none of his patients had this problem five weeks after surgery. He asked if I have a metabolic condition, but I was not sure how to respond. The standard recommendation is another surgery, although I am hesitant. Another surgery so soon would increase the likelihood of an infection and might delay nerve healing. My pectoral muscles might heal if I give them the proper time, support, and the right exercises.

My plan is working better than anticipated. To create proper placement I reposition the implant over the incision as frequently as necessary while lying down. To support the implant, and with the intent of preventing further stretching, I initially resorted to the fitted binding recommended after each surgery. When the binding got uncomfortable (due to my hypersensitive skin) I switched to a soft, well-fitted bra day and night, and for consistency I used the same type of support. Since I can do so little otherwise, I started to at least flex my pectoral muscles on a regular basis. Although initially those muscles were very weak—instead of moving in unison, they would actually quiver. Five weeks later constant support is still necessary, though not as tightly, and I can again place my arms above my shoulders. Even though the problem happened almost every hour for the first two days, the last time was two weeks ago.

The final chapter of this complication has not been written. Surgery might be needed. I'm just willing to give my body a chance to heal, and at least for now, it seems to be working. Surprisingly, the frequent support has provided a mold for my skin and muscles to settle around the implants. Even my plastic surgeon was impressed. My symmetry is atypical, although he is not sure the constant support has played a role.

⊂⊃∞⊙

Implant Infection Information

November 9th-11th

I had another scary experience last week. One morning my left reconstructed breast was noticeably swollen, very red, and quite warm to the touch. It was not painful but I still panicked. I went to see my plastic surgeon that day, even though I was not scheduled to see him for two months. The worst-case scenario was on my mind—an implant infection. I was relieved. An implant infection this far after surgery is unlikely. If it happens, it's usually from another infection, but since I had not been ill that too was unlikely.

Statistics on mastectomy infections are difficult to pin down. Each woman treated for breast cancer undergoes such different treatments. Those include surgeries with or without radiation, chemotherapy prior to or after surgery, and some women have other health conditions. Though generally, mastectomies with no reconstruction hold the lowest rate at 4%, tissue-graft reconstructions have approximately a 7% risk, and mastectomies with implant reconstructions have the highest incidence at 12% [23]. My plastic surgeon explained how, due to the additional healing challenges, surgeries that combine a reconstruction and a mastectomy can create an infection-prone environment. He reminded me that the risk of an infection increases when surgeries are too close to one another, or if healing is not complete.

We explored other possibilities. Increased circulation to the area, the added binding, or the allodynia could be causing the redness. Lymphedema or an irritation from my over-the-counter sports cream could be responsible. We made sure my temperature was not elevated. If it had been, antibiotics would have been unavoidable. He still wrote a prescription for an antibiotic, even though he does not believe they should be taken unnecessarily. However, the redness and the swelling were undeniable.

After filling the prescription I tried to determine what prompted the problem. An infection for no apparent reason seemed to contradict my sense of progress, and my ability to retain the implants in the long run. I was hopeful. Even though they gradually recurred when I got up, the redness and the warmth diminished when I lay down. Had it been an infection, the redness would not have changed with gravity. The redness is on the left side—the one with the greatest nerve discomfort, and where the frozen shoulder occurred—which means I stretch it often, but the fitted bra to control the implant migration could be causing compression. I now loosen my clothes before stretching. Even if this is the culprit, compression and redness were still better than surgery to reposition the implant.

Deodorant seems to increase the nerve discomfort near my left axilla. I removed and reapplied the four different types in our house and interestingly, those with less aluminum were more comfortable. I don't know anything about aluminum. It might not have caused the redness, though just in case, I've switched to a much less effective aluminum-free product.

Preventive measures could prevent implant infections. Avoiding cuts in the kitchen, skipping cuticle removal during manicures, and wearing gloves while gardening should all be considered. Some plastic surgeons recommend antibiotics for procedures such as dental surgeries, but others reserve them for an active implant infection. Removing the implant and restarting the reconstruction at a later date might be necessary if an antibiotic can't resolve an implant infection.

I'm not sure what prompted the problem, but it is no longer present. The infection fright made me appreciate my progress and my new body, imperfect as both might be. Perhaps that is the lesson; accept my new body with all of its discomforts and shortcomings. The old adage is true. *We don't know what we have until we lose it*, or luckily in this case, almost lost it.

⚬⚬⚬

PAIN AFFECTING QUALITY OF LIFE

November 14th

From our balcony I have a perfect beach view of this unseasonably warm, cloudless day—a sharp contrast to my internal environment. I cannot relate. I feel completely detached. We are finally on a trip. Our need to relax and reconnect is suddenly more important than my few predictable comforts at home. After I packed several pillows, and my few bearable shirts, we drove to this gorgeous resort, one of our favorite destinations. This getaway seems necessary for Sandy, but for me it has been a painful reminder—I have many rehabilitative hurdles to conquer.

Unexpectedly, I am comparing this trip to previous ones, from the perspective of how I look and feel. Typically I would be taking long walks and sitting comfortably at the beach. I would not be readjusting shirts or tucking small pillows under my left arm to lessen the nerve pain that results, when anything touches my torso. We also ventured to our favorite outdoor mall, but even though we were there for two hours, I could not find *any* comfortable tops. It was a cool day and many women were wearing long sleeves, though they had no idea how lucky they were; they were warm without discomfort. At least the credit card bill will be low.

The resort's gym was also disappointing. The mirror visual confirmed that I have lost a lot of muscle definition throughout my body in just a few months. The lack of fat on my legs is as concerning as the unwanted 10-pound weight loss, a combination that makes me look way too thin. Even the reflection of my bust-line seemed unfamiliar; in fact, I hardly recognized myself. Most people think I'm healthy because I'm so thin. I neither look nor feel healthy; I look and feel weak. There I stood, in front of the machines I could not even touch, I was that afraid of worsening all of the pain. I walked, though after just 10 minutes I was exhausted. Not knowing how long these limitations will last or how long I will be in pain is very upsetting. Besides, this is not the me I was comfortable or familiar with, which is also depressing.

The saddest thing is how our intimacy has been affected. For several months it has hurt to be touched, and it has been painful to lie down in every position. We used to be the type of couple who would often walk with our arms around each other just to take our dog for a walk, though even that has been difficult. It is not only the weight of my arms that feels uncomfortable, so does the weight of Sandy's hands on most of my upper body—it is unbearable. Our forced distance has been isolating and feels unfair. We are wounded. This is when we need each other the most. I am beginning to see why some marriages with weak bonds prior to cancer end up in divorce. I am not afraid of that happening, even now our bond seems strong. Although, as we slowly try to bridge our distance, I realize how pronounced it has been, and again, how different this trip could have been.

There is an upside, an important one. Assuming it won't hurt, I am not afraid of putting on a bathing suit or a bikini. Most would conclude I had plastic surgery for cosmetic reasons. Yes, my nipple-sparing mastectomy and my reconstruction are up for the challenge.

As this day unfolds, I'll try to redirect my thoughts so that this idyllic setting can fill my soul and nourish my spirit. Things *will* improve. Progress has been taking place. I can start by appreciating the loyal man at my side—his experience has not been an easy one this year. Above all I'll try to enjoy the memories of this amazing place, instead of feeling saddened by them.

◌◌◌

An Insurance Thanksgiving Sentiment

November 26th

It is the day after Thanksgiving and our refrigerator is still filled with the remnants of that wonderful meal. As I quietly enjoy my fall decorations for one more day, the memory of yesterday's celebration still lingers. The main sense is how different this Thanksgiving felt from all others. Not just because of the emotional roller coaster it triggered within me, but because my limitations were obvious to every person at our Thanksgiving table.

There was a question haunting me from the moment I opened my eyes and it seemed important to answer it before tackling the tasks that needed attention. I had to figure out the *main* reason, in the past twelve months, for which I should give thanks. I thought being cancer-free or being alive would have been the obvious response; neither was, not even close. I am grateful for having good health insurance. Without insurance we would have been responsible for the entire bill, not just the reduced amount our insurance company paid. With a plan requiring us to pay 20% of the bill, my treatment options would have also been limited.

Lack of insurance might have affected every aspect of my care. Had I been uninsured, finances would have discouraged an ultrasound, a biopsy, and an MRI. Even under those circumstances my cancer would have been diagnosed, although at a later date, and possibly at a later stage. Since it was already so close, a time delay might have caused the cancer to spread to the lymph nodes. Without insurance my choice of specialists would've been quite different, even at my early stage. The BRAC analysis, which made Nicole's genetic inheritance less concerning, might have also been impossible. Two reconstructive surgeries in a year such as this one would have been downright unaffordable after all of the mentioned expenses. The same could be said of the Oncotype DX, which kept me from receiving chemotherapy and an aromatase inhibitor. Health, and possibly longevity, seems reserved for the insured, particularly the well insured, although I am not sure why I happen to be in that lucky category, when so many others are not.

Most Thanksgiving celebrations take place in our home for convenience sake and this year was no exception. The arrangement was questioned, but I insisted. Hosting Thanksgiving provided a sense of continuity, although I had to accept assistance. I had no choice. My inability to mash potatoes, lift heavy pots, move the turkey, or reposition food trays, proved that my journey is far from over. Everyone was happy to help. We did not let that spoil the day. Those extra helping hands made it clear that I am also blessed with good emotional insurance, also not universal.

Yes, I feel lucky, very lucky, for the benefits adequate health insurance quite literally afforded me last year, but many cannot say the same. With broader access to health care, more women could be diagnosed earlier, and they would receive more effective treatment. Those breast cancer survivors would then experience what I did on this now-memorable Thanksgiving Day: they could enjoy the Thanksgiving blessing without fearing it might be the last.

⤳⤳⤳

DRESSING WITH NERVE PAIN

December 12th-15th

Winter temperatures have officially descended upon the state of Florida, and I might be the only Floridian who is unhappy with that development. Cool temperatures require sleeves, and wearing sleeves is very, very, uncomfortable. After experiencing limited comfort without them, pain with sleeves is suddenly more difficult to accept.

My disappointment goes beyond my dressing difficulties; I am frustrated at how poorly I am handling this new challenge. I am very upset. I have experienced all seasons without dressing as I usually do, and even though it sounds petty in the face of breast cancer, I miss the ability to express myself through clothing.

Out of necessity, I've returned to the mostly futile and always uncomfortable task of trying to shop for shirts. Shifting clothes is painful, carrying even a small bag is uncomfortable, and I can wear almost nothing available. To make sure shirts pass the comfort test for more than an hour at a time, I wear them at home while keeping the tags on. That makes the now familiar step of returning most of them less difficult.

My inability to find tops in stores or catalogs intended for breast cancer patients is disappointing. Though thanks to my teenage daughter, I've realized that teen stores carry spaghetti-strap shirts all year long. The slightly more comfortable, trendier shirts, with soft fabrics and oversized sleeves, can also be found there. Finding tops with soft fabrics such as silk, thin-brushed cotton, rayon, and soft polyesters lacking seams around the shoulders can translate into less discomfort, at least for a short period of time. Although not all items fitting that description are bearable, and I dislike the few items that are tolerable. Disregarding color and attractiveness can, however, be worthwhile. After exhaustive searches, I now own two jackets that can be worn for approximately an hour at a time. Due to their thinness and their three-quarter sleeves they are not very warm, though that is probably what makes them less uncomfortable.

I missed my best opportunity to ask for a pain specialist referral. At a follow-up appointment I was in a tolerable level of discomfort without sleeves, which led me to believe that more pain relief was around the corner. That is not the case. After many phone calls I finally obtained what seems to be a good referral on January 19th—a lifetime away. In the meantime, and thanks to a friend, I tried a topical ointment with a mixture of *Lidocaine* and *Prilocaine*. That seemed like the answer for a few days, but with repeated use my skin looked and felt as if it had been rubbed with sandpaper. The next suggestion was a mixture of *Ketamine* and *Amitriptyline*. Unfortunately my pain became more intense and traveled down my left arm.

Since leaving home limits my ability to change shirts frequently, I am getting more and more isolated as the weather turns colder. On a particularly uncomfortable day I change shirts every twenty minutes. Keeping the house warm has also been necessary. Indoors I am still wearing summer shirts, although I am not looking forward to our heating bill.

To stay warm I wear atypical and sometimes unseasonal combinations. Most days I wear one or two spaghetti-strap shirts, along with one or two of my large-sleeved jackets, depending on the temperature factor. If I must go out, I try to limit the outing to no more than a couple of hours. I also pack several shirts, just like I did when my children were toddlers. To keep the sleeves from touching the back of my arms, I throw a large jacket over my shoulders without using the sleeves. Jackets with a tie or a button at the collar keep the jacket from falling off my shoulders. If it is very cold and wearing sleeves is unavoidable, I reserve them for very short distances, such as between the car and a building. The discomfort and the intensity increase within a short period of time.

Other changes have been necessary. I placed the few items that I can wear in one specific section of my closet. Since there is so little to choose from, getting dressed with such few choices can be easier. The key is to stay focused on what I *can* wear rather than what I cannot. I took some of the large shirts in at the waist and left their large sleeves intact, though even then, those are only tolerable for short periods of time. Wearing soft shawls sometimes helps, although they are not very warm or practical, they get in the way if I am cooking or performing other chores. Humor helps. I've joked about how my only winter statement is a darker color, not long sleeves. Another strategy worth practicing is to focus on getting by one day at a time, without panicking about the possibility of permanent pain.

Remembering what is good in my life does not always work. These days, my mood tends to rise and fall along with the thermostat readings. In every sense of the word, winter has never felt so cold. But it is good to live in a state known for registering temperatures above 70 degrees in the month of December. When the temperature increases, I can see light at the end of my lengthy tunnel. The warm days and the comfort from the limited clothing remind me that all of this is only temporary.

⚬⚭⚬

DELAYED MOURNING

December 18th

There might be another explanation for my less-than-positive outlook. Now that I am done with doctors' appointments, diagnostic procedures, and since my family is no longer worried, I can mourn the cancer experience for myself.

How could I have been so naïve? Why did I believe I would not hit an emotional brick wall at some point? I should be glad it did not happen before, that would've been overwhelming. This feels like posttraumatic stress. My mourning is surfacing afterwards, under less stressful circumstances. I don't know why I'm surprised or disappointed. I recall similar reactions.

Just as I am starting to mourn, my family and friends want me to go back to being my old self. I wish I could, but I can't. What's more, I am not sure I can, I feel so different. Some long-term friends and family members promised to always listen, except lately even they seem to prefer more upbeat subjects. I understand. We are in the midst of the holidays, why would they want to talk about breast cancer? No, I cannot avoid breast cancer thoughts. My nerve discomfort, my clothing limitations, the need to constantly stretch, and my arm weaknesses are constant reminders, although for their sake, I am trying to leave my family out of the loop.

I finally want to speak with other survivors about their experiences. I've searched for personal accounts and have gone to some blogs, though I prefer face-to-face discussions. Tatiana is a good sounding board, although she has her own mountains to climb. She just went back to surgery for her permanent implants after six months of her own eventful reconstruction. I should not put any more stress on her. What I really need is a support group. I will search for one next year when I have more time; for now, journaling will have to suffice.

I am trying to lower my stress in ways I can control. I am exercising in my limited manner, I try to meditate frequently, and I usually keep a balanced diet. I try to rest through my discomfort and I ask for help with difficult chores. Lowering my expectations in the fashion and the housekeeping department are also necessary, but they are not enough. Finding time to mourn seems important, a concept I learned from one of my favorite books: *Tuesdays with Morrie*. When necessary, professor Morrie grieved his impending death for a limited period in the morning, then focused on what was still good in his life for the rest of the day [4].

If I can find hidden lessons now, I might have more appreciation for future experiences. I keep remembering what I've often told our children; just like rainbows, life would not be the same without the color blue. The teachings of the Dalai Lama also seem appropriate; he believes difficult situations and emotions are simply part of life, the difference lies in how we respond [72]. I seem to be undergoing a metamorphosis through all of this physical and emotional pain, not unlike a caterpillar goes through before becoming a butterfly.

⸎

LYMPHEDEMA AND COPING WITH STRENGTH DEFICITS

December 20th-21st

It can no longer be ignored. My long walks are causing left arm and chest discomfort, as uncomfortable as a couple of months ago. Even though I am hoping it is temporary, lymphedema is now undeniable. The lymphedema is mild. Visibly neither arm is larger, and the pins-and-needle sensation, along with the swelling that makes the rings on my left hand feel tight, subsides after a couple of hours. The problem is less noticeable when I walk on an indoor treadmill, assuming I rest my arms on the side bars. I will miss my walks outside. It took a while to build up the exercise tolerance and they were a wonderful outlet.

I am trying to avoid a lymphedema sleeve. Compression and nerve pain have the potential to be a very painful combination. Instead, I've been consistent with my lymphedema-prevention exercises. I am also avoiding triggering activities, such as lifting heavy objects.

When I overtire my left arm, the discomfort is obvious for hours or for days at a time. The pain can be triggered by overreaching, overstretching, or when I use that arm in a repetitive manner. In those instances the sharp pain is immediate, although swelling is not noticeable. As this example illustrates, I have to concentrate on every move I make. For three days I was able to do light chores with limited discomfort, but then last night I tried to close a high curtain with my left arm. The failed attempt brought the familiar tightness under and around the upper portion of that arm. Soon the pain radiated to the left side of my neck and shoulder, as it usually does. If history repeats itself, I'll have to choose between being cold and being in pain. If I am careful most of the discomfort will pass by the end of the week, but avoiding activities will not restore my strength. On the other hand, it is winter—the main priority is warmth—I should avoid new efforts and limit activities to those that have proven comfortable. Ignoring either guideline can set me back for days.

Predetermining how I am going to tackle each and every task can limit pain. To engage my legs, it is always better to stoop down before lifting an object. For most tasks it is better to use only my right arm. Using both arms is sometimes possible, assuming I keep most of the weight on the right side. For light tasks, such as opening a cabinet door, I can finally use only my left arm, and I take advantage of every light-mobility opportunity to strengthen that weak limb. As expected, those options don't always suffice. At times I have to swallow my pride and request help from anyone, including strangers. My family is quite confused. On some days I need minimal assistance, while on others I require a lot more. I understand. I too am confused.

❧

2010

Cancer & New Year's Resolutions

January 1st

It is good to start a new year, even though I did not want to be part of a big celebration last night. Instead, Neil and I watched movies and talked. He did not want me to be alone, a gesture I will not forget. A couple of neighbors invited us to celebrate New Year's Eve with a little more flare. They knew I would be glad to bid farewell to this past year. I declined. I wanted to be in safe territory in case I became emotional. Saying good-bye to last year was after all a personal matter.

I used to be the kind of person who made New Year's resolutions and tried hard to abide by them, but I cannot do that this year. I am only asking for the emotional and the physical strength to handle whatever is in store for me. Cancer reminded me that anything can happen at any time, even when we are making plans that might never come true. At least for now, the realization has made New Year's resolutions pointless.

That is not all. Another outlook is evident today because of my habit of looking into the future on New Year's Day. A few months ago Nicole expressed that after cancer everything revolved around me. She was referring to people asking about me, cooking for me, and doing things for me. She went from being the center of our world to watching me become the focus. Her comment applies—it was truer than either of us could have grasped at the time—I suddenly want to honor what is important for me. I want my legacy to be about more than being a mother and about more than being a wife. I have enjoyed those roles immensely. I have no regrets, none, period. No matter what else I do with my life, being a mother will always be *the* most important thing I have ever done; but now, I need to contribute beyond my local volunteering.

I've been developing an interest in breast cancer causes. In many ways I feel like I have been, and continue to be, in training for that very purpose. But all of that will have to wait until much, much, later. As I start this year, I have to find a way to diminish the constant pain, and I need to regain some strength.

WEAKNESS INTERFERING WITH RESPONSIBILITIES

January 14th

Clearly, I knew this year would hold some surprises, I just did not realize they would come this soon. Even though careful, mindful mobility created a little more comfort, all of that changed a few days ago when my mother fell. She broke her ankle in several locations. Extensive surgery was necessary, and by extension, she now requires frequent assistance. The unwelcome situation, and the strain of pushing her in a wheelchair, increased all of my pain on a permanent basis.

I am not just a poor caretaker in pain—I am an inadequate family member. I was forced to rule out the possibility of her staying in our home, which under different circumstances would have been the most practical arrangement for all parties involved. My refusal seems wrong on the surface, but it makes sense from a broader perspective. Can I be a caretaker if I am still having trouble holding a book, emptying my dishwasher, and cutting vegetables for dinner?

Feeling essentially handicapped makes challenging situations more difficult. My pain and weakness are very disruptive. Even though I am not sure how the goal can be accomplished, addressing my strength deficits is extremely important. There is also no time for support groups. My grieving will have to be delayed.

❧

PAIN SPECIALIST CONSULT

January 22nd

The long-awaited appointment with the pain specialist finally took place. I was glad. I am definitely ready to take the next step, although I was afraid to hear the words *permanent pain*. I was not sure how hearing the sentence would affect my morale.

A month long search for the right referral, and the six week wait for the appointment were worth the hassle. He not only came highly regarded, he also has neurological training and a surgical background, an appropriate combination if an invasive procedure is needed.

Credentials aside, his warm personality and his conservative approach impressed me the most. He felt that since I've been through enough invasive pro-cedures lately, it would be premature to contemplate nerve blocks or trigger point injections. I underwent several tests to check my strength, reflexes, sensation, and then I had a series of X-rays. I learned that nerve endings heal very slowly; he confirmed they usually heal at approximately 1 millimeter per month.

Pharmaceuticals might be helpful. He suggested I try oral Neurontin, even though I told him it makes me feel dizzy at the lowest dose. To sleep off the dizziness he suggested I take the same amount at bedtime, and so that my body can adjust gradually, the dose should be tripled over several weeks. He suggested I apply a Lidocaine patch at the crease in the back of my left arm, although I am hesitant. According to the nurse it cannot be cut from its large size. The plastic or paper from the patch might cause even more discomfort since not even soft fabrics can be tolerated in that area. Besides, Lidocaine might again irritate my skin, which my physician husband says is not uncommon.

As far as my left arm strength, pain, and tightness issues, he feels that a muscular complication is prolonging my pain. He prescribed a muscle relaxant and referred to the syndrome as a *myofascial dysfunction*. He would like to focus on specific stretches and strengthening exercises, all of which will start in physical therapy next week.

My progress might continue, possibly into a full recovery. That was so good to hear! After such a long time, I was starting to fear permanent nerve and muscular pain. It is exciting to have a plan from a professional who seems to understand what is wrong with me, and without the term *permanent nerve damage* as part of that description.

❦

ARTICLE SHEDS LIGHT ON PAIN SYNDROME

January 24th-25th

Since myofascial dysfunction is now part of my medical history, I researched it shortly after the appointment with the pain specialist. My search produced limited, though fairly productive, results. I found "Barriers to Rehabilitation Following Surgery for Primary Breast Cancer," published in the *Journal of Surgical Oncology* in 2007, by Dr. Andrea L. Cheville, M.D., and Dr. Julia Tchou, M.D. [31].

I unearthed a treasure. The article perfectly describes my experiences. It provides important information on *myofascial dysfunctions, lymphedema,* and *frozen shoulders*. It also addresses post-mastectomy syndrome, which some experts call *post breast therapy pain syndrome*, since it can also occur after breast-conservation surgery. I learned about the one complication in the article I did not experience: *axillary web syndrome*, which happens when lymph cords swell and get hard after losing the lymph nodes that typically drain them. I was surprised to learn that lymphedema can worsen allodynia and muscular dysfunctions. On the upside, mild lymphedema episodes improve with time and with manual drainage techniques, which I am performing daily.

To prevent unnecessary procedures, delay treatment, and avoid further injury, additional cancer rehabilitation training is needed. Physical therapy is effective in some facilities, but not in all. Follow-up care can also be challenging, even when a proper diagnosis is made. Conflicting work schedules, lack of nearby services, insufficient patient cooperation, or inadequate insurance coverage can all interfere [31]. I might be one of the lucky ones. I was diagnosed by someone who seems to understand breast cancer complications. I also have adequate health insurance and available time. Although I wonder how others, lacking so many resources, would fare under similar circumstances.

❦

EXPLANATIONS FOR PROLONGED PAIN

February 8th-13th

It might seem surprising, but I am not upset about the addition to my medical repertoire, not at all. The physical therapy is not invasive, and the diagnosis would explain why I've been unable to progress. Going through physical therapy might not only provide pain relief, it might offer strength as a welcome bonus. I might even be able to wear sleeves in the near future, but I should not get ahead of myself just yet.

Although, the physical therapy lingo is challenging; I'm not familiar with muscle names in the upper arms, back, and neck, or with their intended functions, therefore I'm having trouble understanding easily shared explanations. From what I've been able to gather, as far as breast cancer patients are concerned, the term myofascial dysfunction describes abnormal movements or muscular traumas from surgery, pain, nerve disruptions, radiation, or from reconstruction weight burdens, such as implants.

When weaker muscles cannot perform they are *under-functioning,* which can make surrounding muscles *overcompensate,* or work harder than they should. In other words, muscular problems might not remain isolated. *Surrounding* muscles might pull, stretch, and work in unnatural patterns, a combination that can become a vicious cycle. Over time muscle-to-muscle size ratios are altered, and that causes even more asymmetry. Those patterns are difficult to reverse, cause pain, and result in additional injury.

It seems as though my myofascial dysfunction involves muscles beyond my upper arm; it extends into that side of my back, shoulder, and neck. Some of those muscles have minimal strength, have atrophied, and have shortened. Therefore those muscles need to be stretched, strengthened, and repositioned. It also seems that other muscles have been overcompensating, have overdeveloped, and are very tight. That is why those muscles need to be massaged, rested, and retrained to not do so much.

My limited awareness is making it difficult to understand why I need to perform certain movements, although some make sense from the symptoms I've been experiencing. My very smart therapist described how there are two muscles that wrap around the upper arm; one around the *front*, and the other towards the back *underneath* that same location. Due to my lack of sensation and weakness, those muscles tightened and shortened over partially atrophied muscles. That is why, for months, I've been sensing a tourniquet sensation in the upper part of my left arm when I reach, pull, or press. Even more exciting is the possibility that those wraparound muscles might be interfering with lymphatic drainage and compressing nerves. Blocked lymph drainage, from muscular tightness, could be contributing to the pain and swelling when I take long walks. Those are all good news, seemingly unrelated problems might improve.

There is another problem that now makes sense. Three months ago I developed constant left-sided neck discomfort that worsens when I sit or lie down. Apparently some of my neck muscles shortened, as my left shoulder got displaced in forward manner. Months of keeping my left arm slightly up and away from my torso, to lessen the underarm nerve discomfort, has not helped this situation. The discomfort has caused headaches and jaw pain, which might explain why my dentist claims I crushed a tooth on that side. Wow! To encourage the realignment I will have to maintain good posture, position my arms close to my torso, and keep my shoulders rolled back. Those poses will be challenging, they are so painful.

I am still hoping these setbacks are temporary, but I am starting to wonder how much comfort and strength I'll eventually regain. The outcome of this situation, like so many others in the past year, is an unknown I simply have to accept, even though I have to do what I can to improve the outcome.

Explanations are a good place to start. It is good to know that something very specific, though difficult, can be attempted. A short-lived sense of relief is a step in the right direction, although this will not get treated overnight. I am again relying on frequent meditations, relaxation periods, and self-massages, especially at night. Sleep has been challenging. The discomfort around the top of my left arm goes away with physical therapy massages, but it returns with activities such as cooking and driving. Some pain is expected to increase when we try to strengthen my weakest muscles. Perhaps Jane Fonda was right with her *no-pain-no-gain* mantra.

⚜️

Energy Medicine & Generational Pain

Feb 27th-March 3rd

The last few weeks have been amazingly healing and incredibly surreal, so much so that I do not know where to start my narration. Perhaps I can begin with an update. These days the discomfort to the front of my left arm is more difficult to trigger, it is easier to manage, and that arm appears to have a little more strength.

Physical therapy seems to be addressing left arm and shoulder muscular imbalances, but it was never intended to lessen the nerve sensitivity that plagues my entire chest and the back of my left upper arm. Neurontin, prescribed in January, was prescribed for that purpose. Many people tolerate the medicine with few side effects and in high doses. I could not. Even at half of the lowest dose it gave me a severe headache, made it impossible to sleep, and it made me feel dizzy and depressed. Since I've already tried several other pharmaceuticals, and I am concerned about invasive procedures, the options felt limited, although my ongoing discomfort was starting to weaken that resolve.

At this point I must forewarn that my tale is about to become atypical and unusual, perhaps significantly so. It all started a few weeks ago when we attended a party. There I was given a referral for a psychologist proficient in a type of energy medicine called *Body Talk*. I liked the idea of a reliable psychologist right away—I definitely need help in the emotional department.

My discomfort has been making me a little desperate, although that is not the only reason I took the phone number. While in New Hampshire for Andrew's graduation I experienced the positive effects of energy medicine. At the time I chose a therapeutic massage, the only one that could be performed without lying on my stomach. Unbeknownst to me, it was not a traditional massage. I later realized it resembled a technique called *Reiki*. With minimal guidance on my part, the massage therapist relieved some of my pain by simply placing her hands over my most painful areas. She said that "pain has a warmer feel to it." The experience left me curious about energy medicine; I obtained noticeable, though temporary, relief. My mind could not comprehend how or why it had worked, but having less pain allowed me to enjoy that important weekend.

Energy medicine is based on Chinese medicine principles. The Chinese believe that our bodies have energy fields with specific paths, and when those fields are out of balance or the paths are blocked, disease or difficulties with healing can result. There are different types of energy medicine, though Body Talk claims to enhance communication between mind and body, and by extension innate healing. Clearly, that is a very simple explanation for an approach so different from traditional medicine, but the undeniable relief from the Reiki experience prompted a search for an energy medicine practitioner. I did not want just anybody. I wanted an impressive word-of-mouth referral from a trusted source, and preferably for someone with an impressive résumé. It took nearly eight months, but I finally got the referral at a birthday party last month.

At any rate, the events that have been taking place appear as difficult to explain as they have been to experience, and yet I will try to do just that. I want to stay true to a promise. I vowed to document my breast cancer experience with complete honesty and in its entirety.

On the first appointment a month ago, I noticed that the therapist is a soft-spoken, kind, quick-witted middle-age woman, who can probably make anyone relax. She asked if I knew how Body Talk works. I did not. She replied that to some extent neither did she, but that some people find it life altering. I lay on what appeared to be a massage table, as she placed one of her hands on my stomach and the other over my right wrist. She remained in silence, interrupting only to inquire about my marital status and ethnicity.

Then she stated that the core of my pain had been passed from mother to daughter for four generations, and it was influencing my emotions and thoughts. She explained that she could not tell me what to do, but I would know what to do. I confirmed her suspicions. Friction between my mother and I has been the norm for years. There were greater difficulties between her and her deceased mother, and it all started with my grandmother's mother—four generations of mothers and daughters. I shared that therapy, reading, and careful parenting on my part, kept Nicole from being part of that generational chain. The session was briefer than anticipated. It only lasted 30 to 40 minutes. As I began the lengthy drive through the country roads between her office and our home, I wondered if the exercise had been in vain. It was a beautiful spring day and I was in unusually high spirits, but that changed within minutes. I was suddenly overcome by grief—my grandmother's. I kept repeating *I am so sorry, Grandma, I never knew*.

I decided to go see my mother, the one person who might understand what I was experiencing. I was not sure what I was going to say. Discussions about negative family events have never been her strongest point. I often wondered why, at the age of five, I was made to choose between my parents when they divorced. Why did I spend third grade in a convent and a year in a different part of the country, where I was sexually abused by someone we all respected?

Our childhood had many other challenges. After the divorce we moved multiple times to keep my father from finding us, a constant uprooting that limited childhood friends. Before my 13th birthday my mother married an American. While rather strongly suggesting that we neither mention nor contact our own living father, my stepfather demanded we call him "dad" on the day we met. He was also an alcoholic and a molester who became belligerent at a moment's notice.

The language barrier prevented schoolwork or refuge in my beloved books, and I turned to the only teens who seemed to understand me: problem kids. Anger, rebelliousness, drugs, alcohol, and home avoidance became the norm. Our American schools lacked language transition programs and out of frustration I quit school in the middle of my sophomore year. My run away status for nearly 12 months had no legal repercussions, but that was nothing short of miraculous.

Even though I returned when my stepfather left, the mother-to-daughter bond was fractured. We called many truces over the years, but since we never observed clear, reasonable boundaries, the truces did not last. Neither of us could possibly know that the status quo would change with a single conversation on that Tuesday afternoon, after my first Body Talk session.

It all started when my grandmother was born. She was rejected by her mother, because her infant skin color was darker than her siblings'. The motherly disdain was very pronounced—my great-grandfather took her on his work-related journeys when she was just a toddler. My grandmother was soon forced to live with distant relatives while her mother, father, and siblings, carried on with normal family life. My grandmother became a maid in those households. In Colombia, during the mid-1920s and early 1930s, that arrangement was nothing short of an insult for a middle-class girl with an intact family. When my grandmother was a young teen her mother died. She thought she could finally live with her beloved father, but unrelated events prevented the reunion. My grandmother never experienced her family's love.

A few years later my grandmother's relatively new marriage failed, although my grandfather made his own contribution. He lost their respectable financial assets, including their home, in one night's worth of gambling, when their three daughters were still under the age of five. He moved in with his wealthy parents, who decided to let their daughter-in-law and her three young daughters fend for themselves. The result of so much drama—difficult to believe in a soap opera— was that my grandmother raised her three girls physically and financially alone. After so much disillusionment my grandmother became a stern, heavy-handed woman, with her three daughters and with her grandchildren.

When she was just 15 years old my mother sought to escape by marrying a man she did not know well who was 20 years her senior—my father. As expected, my parents' marriage was another relationship doomed to fail, long before it began. His life experiences ensured his own difficulties as a husband, and as a father. He was the only live-in son of a bitter, unmarried woman, who boycotted the relationship from the start.

The mother-to-daughter discord did its share of damage in other branches of our family. There are more stories than I will ever know or could possibly reiterate. These only give a *sense* of the many lives that were eventually touched by my great-grandmother's disdain.

When I observed how frail my mother looked in her wheelchair from her broken ankle, I understood that receiving such limited affection caused multiple difficulties when my mother and my grandmother became parents. Without premeditation I uttered the words I thought I would never be able to articulate: "I forgive you." I did it on impulse, but also because I sensed Grandma needed the mother-to-daughter discord to finally end. For the first time, in a long time, we were relating to one another without being defensive of every word and of every imagined undertone. She could see my pain, just like I was seeing hers, then something clicked between us and we embraced in tears.

Needless to say that evening I sensed multiple emotions, although those paled by comparison to the ones I experienced throughout the night and the following morning. Within a couple of hours I began to dream that beings of light were coming in and out of my chest. I somehow understood they were souls who had been negatively affected by the four generations of mothers and daughters. All of them seemed to be lessening their pain by coming in contact with me, and each was taking a little of mine as they passed. The process was neither painful nor difficult, at least not until I sensed one of them was my grandfather's soul. His pain left me out of breath. I got up to search for my inhaler.

Up until that point I could have rationalized the entire experience as a difficult and symbolic dream, but that possibility ended when I got up. Through the dim bathroom lighting I was able to smell him, see him, and I even heard him speak to me. He had a musty smell as if he had been perspiring from a long walk outdoors, which I know he loved to do. He was wearing a dark suit and a partially unbuttoned white shirt. His eyes were dark and deeply set, but the main thing I noticed about them was how they sparkled in the dark. His face was tanned, rugged, and his well-ingrained wrinkles framed his half-grin. Seeing him in such vivid detail was particularly difficult to believe; I had only seen him a handful of times before the age of five. Then he simply said "miija." He said it so slowly that he actually dragged the word into a loving whisper. At that moment I sensed his love. It seemed to embrace me, but then he was gone. That word is a merging of the Spanish words *mi* and *hija*—it means *my daughter*. My mother and aunt have since confirmed that when he spoke with them, he frequently used the expression.

The unusual experiences did not end that night. I had more atypical dreams. In one dream I was in surgery being repaired, in another I was dancing in light. In one vivid dream I spoke with my grandmother. I told her how wonderful Nicole is. I explained that she is free to love and live her life as she chooses, I happily described how well we get along, and I let her know that Nicole was named after her. Within ten days of the initial episode, the extreme level of sensitivity that plagued my entire chest, to the point of having lace and jewelry hurt, subsided by close to 60%. That joy was short lived. It was replaced by the deep sadness that has been unleashed by various consultations, where the therapist combines counseling with Body Talk.

Many things have surfaced, including the loss of our first baby, the lack of a father figure, and the death of my grandmother. In my life, her role was that of a parent. The suicide and premature deaths of more friends than I care to name, my inability to forgive the abuse, my sense of loneliness as a child, and of course the emotional, and the physical, pain of my breast cancer have also emerged. One by one, each and every traumatic event has presented itself. They all want to be properly mourned for as long as it takes. Since I can never predict when the sadness will surface, I've become a hermit.

I am physically and emotionally drained. These emotions have taken me by surprise, have been overwhelming, and have unleashed an ocean of tears. This feels like *the* emotional catharsis of my life. Perhaps the tip of this iceberg was trying to emerge in December when I was starting to feel depressed. It does feel like I have been accumulating grief for decades; although to my amazement, it is now being released through this unusual process. This catharsis is somehow necessary. The healing feels psychological, spiritual, and also physical.

⁂

PHYSICAL THERAPY COUNTERPRODUCTIVE

March 11th

A few days ago, on February 29th, I completed three one-hour physical therapy appointments per week over a six-week period, as well as daily recommended exercises. After that the plan called for three weeks of home stretches, weights, and light-band exercises. Then I was to go back to receive the next level of training, a cycle that would continue for as long as necessary.

That was the plan of course, although this plan did not workout as anticipated, as is often the case when we try to predict an outcome. Perhaps the massages I received in therapy are the missing ingredient. The pain is again constant, not just intermittent as was the case during the weeks I attended physical therapy. Although it isn't all bad news; thanks to physical therapy I lost most of the left-upper-arm tourniquet sensation, and I got a better sense of what is causing the pain.

To see if there was something else he could suggest or do, a few days ago I returned to physical therapy. The therapist did several manipulations and placed a large ice pack with an electrical stimulation unit on my shoulder. Except instead of the anticipated relief, the pain increased threefold that night, and for the next two sleepless days. I finally obtained a little relief from ultraviolet heat, a clear indication that the plan is altogether wrong.

Today I reported to the pain specialist that I am not willing to continue with this physical therapy approach. Not only has most of the pain recurred, it is worse than it was before. He is now concerned. Several nerves travel from the side of the neck, towards the shoulder, and into the axilla, but therapy cannot progress if one of them is damaged or compressed. He wants me to try a different muscle relaxant at a low dose. To determine if something else is causing the pain, I need a neck and a thorax MRI. I also received a prescription for a topical cream, not unlike the one I tried a few months ago with limited results. Except this one has 2% of both *Ketamine* and *Amitriptyline,* as opposed to the previous 1% and 2%. The new prescription also has Lidocaine, the very ingredient that caused so much skin irritation, which is why I've decided to retry my previous ointment. Besides, the combination does not have FDA approval, and without insurance the cost of the first ointment is $100 for a narrow two-inch container. He strongly advised I take *Lyrica* to lower my nerve sensitivity. If my nerve pain continues much longer, it could become permanent. Not exactly what I was hoping to hear.

This puzzle has a missing piece. My rehabilitation can't move forward until I find it.

❦

EMOTIONAL & SPIRITUAL UPHEAVAL

March 12th-15th

If I were to say that I am in an emotional state of awe, it would be an understatement. I cannot deny the spiritual significance or the psychological importance of the events of the past few weeks, although the same applies to the experiences before my first surgery. I am trying to avoid rational explanations. They don't work. Besides, my unusual experiences will not fit into any spiritual mold. Since the experiences were so personal in nature, their interpretation should probably occur at that same level. I have to use my heart, not my brain.

I've often wondered if physical, mental, and spiritual healing, can be enhanced by approaches other than traditional ones, although the subject did not have a personal agenda—not until I got cancer. My interest started in the late 1980s when I worked in various intensive care units, and took psychology classes on my days off. I felt like a jealous, distant observer. I witnessed how some of my patients flexed their spiritual muscle to help them cope with extreme grief, physical challenges, loss of loved ones, and even their own deaths. Surprisingly, no spiritual background had the market cornered on its ability to help. The requirement appeared to be as simple as it was unattainable for me—having blind faith.

As I studied him, I had difficulty understanding why Carl Jung gave up working with the giant that was Sigmund Freud in 1913, after a symbolic dream [80]. In time he studied various cultures, religious philosophies, and developed a dream theory. He concluded that we carry *archetypal symbols,* which can reveal themselves in dreams, feelings, or with intuition that can seem life changing [79]. Dr. Jung's courage to stand up for his beliefs at such a time and in such a manner had always impressed me, although until recently, I could not grasp the spiritual meaning behind his theories. I now wonder if generational pain could fall under the archetypal symbol definition.

I am starting to understand some of Dr. Bernie Siegel's messages. In *Peace, Love & Healing,* he talks about the "gifts" that are available to patients who do the emotional and the spiritual work of cancer [147]. In *Love, Medicine, and Miracles,* he asks, "Why did you need the illness?" He believes that we, the cancer patients, must eventually ask that of ourselves, to maximize our emotional and our physical healing [146]. The question was too difficult to entertain after my diagnosis, but a year of unexpected experiences opened the door to healing opportunities. Cancer has been, and continues to be, instrumental for the release of stored emotions, while making me aware of how loved I am. Cancer brought me closer to several family members, including my mother, and it helped me understand our generational pain. Above all, cancer unexpectedly broke down the barriers that were restraining my spirituality.

Even though I had always admired people who felt guided by prayer, I blocked real spirituality from coming into my life. I was way too rational and much too analytical, although for reasons beyond my medical exposure. I thought most of the benefits derived from prayer were psychological. I attributed the sense of euphoria to the believer's focus on a repetitive mantra—similar to the sense of well-being derived from meditation. I also thought trusting things I could not understand or control would suggest weakness on my part, but I could not have been further from the truth.

Yes, I learned to meditate, but only because I understood the physical benefits: meditation can lower blood pressure, slow the heart rate, and diminish oxygen consumption. After years of practicing meditation it had become a pleasant, addictive sensation that reduced stress.

All of that has finally changed. What seems to be working is to simply listen without resistance. I need to accept the insights, but without questioning them on a rational level. In retrospect this process has been evolving since before my diagnosis, and even though I was unaware of the magnitude of its influence, I've been relying on a spiritual compass. The amazing thing is that I've gained so much, and from such simple techniques; from meditative prayer, from staying focused on the joys of the moment, and because I no longer try to control outcomes. Those simple mindsets opened the door to unexpected experiences. When I was diagnosed with breast cancer, and for the first time in my life, I prayed with a sense of urgency, with an open mind, and with a tremendous need to make a connection.

Cancer showed me that other approaches can complement traditional medicine. I've learned that balance (and occasionally healing) between mind, body, and spirit is not only possible, it can sometimes be achieved under extremely stressful circumstances. I am humbled and astounded. What's more, I am grateful.

Life feels more complete. To my amazement, these insights have made my pain and mobility difficulties easier to bear.

❧

CERVICAL COMPRESSION

March 18th

I had to come up with a diagnosis for the constant burning pain two inches below the base of my skull. My next appointment with the pain specialist is not for another five weeks. After research, I believe I am experiencing *cervical compression* (swelling in my spine), as a result of extreme upper-torso muscular tightness.

Different things can be attempted. Avoidance of what is causing the problem is the first, but that cannot happen—the muscle tightness remains. Performing frequent neck stretches, such as tilting the head forward and from side to side for several seconds at a time is one of those recommended motions. Not surprisingly, the movement is tight and limited, which is why I need to pursue it. For muscular relaxation, I started muscle relaxants ten days ago and I frequently massage both neck and shoulders. Massaging the source of the pain worsens the discomfort, but massaging around the area tends to lessen it. I stopped using weights and bands, as suggested in physical therapy, both clearly aggravate the problem. I am also relying on ice to reduce pain and minimize swelling.

Being middle-aged and dealing with conflicting breast cancer detours can be complex. I have to listen to my body and become informed.

❧

PERSONALIZED PAIN MANAGEMENT ATTEMPTS

March 21st

I have been unable to fill the Lyrica prescription. Our insurance company wants a letter explaining why I cannot take Neurontin, which works for many people and is less expensive. I was initially frustrated. I was prepared to take medicine, even though I still have concerns, but the postponement encouraged creative ideas that seem promising.

It all started when I tried to identify which movements increase the pain, so that I can modify or avoid them. With that goal in mind I've been moving in a slower, gentler pace, which is easier to accomplish in water. I've also been relying on a Jacuzzi to lessen muscular tension, but I have to keep heat away from what feels like nerve pain in the back of my neck.

The Ketamine and Amitriptyline ointment is finally helping. Three to five times a day I apply small amounts to the most uncomfortable locations, although not at the base of my skull; it amplifies the cervical compression pain. The results are now effective and immediate, although short lived. They only last about two hours. Maybe the tight muscles at the top of my left arm were keeping the ointment from working, or maybe those nerves had to regenerate before they could benefit. Regardless of the cause, it is good to have nerve pain relief without significant side effects.

I might not start Lyrica if I continue doing this well without it. The medicine was prescribed to reduce nerve pain, and that has unexpectedly lessened in most areas. I will still fill the prescription when it becomes available. The pain specialist planted a fear seed that has already given fruit. When he explained that my pain could become permanent if not soon relieved, I got more involved.

⚜

FIRST SURVIVORSHIP ANNIVERSARY

March 25th-26th

Without hesitation, the 23rd of this month was an important milestone—I became a one-year breast cancer survivor!

The period leading up to that day was challenging. A sense of disappointment seemed to predominate, and not just because physical therapy did not work out as expected. I had set the one-year anniversary as *the* target date for my physical recovery. I had envisioned the day. It was going to be cancer-free *and* pain-free; therefore, the inability to accomplish one of those goals was a letdown. I felt extremely disappointed, and not just because I failed to accomplish one of my intended goals. I still lack a clear sense of direction to start tackling the rest.

Despite their negative contribution, I had been taking the muscle relaxants for a couple of weeks. Except the medicine was making me feel depressed, seemed to help minimally, and it kept me from sleeping, which was particularly problematic. Being so tired kept me from exercising, and under normal circumstances that helps when I feel down. For some reason the sedation also made it impossible to meditate. That had taken away my spiritual guidance and my most effective pain reliever. When I compared the muscle relaxants' limited benefit against the multiple side effects, I understood my body was sending a clear signal: I have to look for nonchemical approaches to ease my pain. I stopped the muscle relaxants on the morning of my one-year anniversary as a symbolic new direction. Just the idea of no longer living under a medicated cloud made me feel hopeful, although also anxious. Without pharmaceuticals or physical therapy, I am stepping into uncertain territory.

My understandable disappointment disappeared by the second half of the day, but only after I allowed a brief trip down sad-memory lane. There I recalled the anxiety that led up to the surgery, the ongoing pain, and the multiple difficulties that followed. The comparison of those more challenging days against my progress, though incomplete, made it clear that life is more difficult without gratitude, and that it feels nearly miraculous when I am able to stay open and positive, even if the prize is more physical discomfort. I am glad to have my appreciation back. I was afraid it had left me for good.

Yes, my second year as a cancer survivor should be a good one, especially since important family events will take place. We will attend Andrew's wedding, Neil's graduation, and two other large family weddings. My one-year anniversary is a new beginning, not the end of my healing. My body's ability to heal is not like the pages of a calendar—it does not run out after twelve months. It is also not like sand in an hourglass, which empties after a limited period of time. I *know* my recovery will continue.

In a roundabout way, my wish did come true. As I started focusing on how much healing has taken place, and when I completely understood that it will continue, the renewed gratitude allowed us to mark my survivorship milestone. We had a celebratory dinner outing and a toast, which became very emotional on my part.

❧

WHY PHYSICAL THERAPY COULD NOT HELP

March 29th-30th

I am determined to overcome my rehabilitative hurdles, but first I must turn back the clock. *How did my muscles become so dysfunctional?* I am specifically looking for information that can explain how rehabilitation should be approached with the *combination* of nerve damage and muscular complications. I believe the problem lies at exactly that juncture. Unfortunately I'm having trouble, other than the verification that both can happen after breast cancer treatments.

I spent last weekend surrounded by anatomy books and rehabilitation infor-mation. I was surprised; I already understand a great deal. My very educated six-week therapist taught me a lot. He was right. My weakest muscles are in my upper arms. Just like many other patients, I developed problems in those areas after surgery.

In order to understand which muscles have atrophied, are the weakest, and need to be strengthened first, I compared how my arms and shoulders are respond-ing to the physical therapy exercises. By doing a manual and a visual side-to-side comparison, I understood which muscles are *supposed* to be moving on the left side, except I learned that some are not moving at all. The portion of my *trapezius* muscle, which runs from the base of my skull and into my left shoulder, has been doing most of the work. In simpler terms, muscles that were already tight got tighter during the six weeks of physical therapy, and some of the ones that were supposed to get stronger got weaker. All of that explains why some muscles are still wasting, why they have minimal strength, and why the physical therapy rou-tine causes pain. I need to find a way to strengthen the right muscles, but without weight-bearing exercises. Lifting as little as one pound tightens the wrong muscles and causes severe pain.

Those clarifications, along with better upper-torso anatomy understanding, paved the way for creative ideas. Those presented themselves as I was contemplat-ing the usual interaction between muscles, nerves, and tendons in the weak and uncomfortable areas. Even though the physical therapy goal was to strengthen and relax the muscles in my upper arms and back, other important muscles were not seen as part of the problem.

Specifically, my pectoral muscles seem weak, tight, and guarded. I started thinking that if a domino effect results when one set of muscles is not working well, then the torso pain, just under my left upper arm, might be from either pec-toral muscle tightness or weakness. When I stretch, move, or lift anything that should involve the pectoral muscles, the pain in that location, and then in other areas, is immediately triggered. Unfortunately the realization came a week after my appointment with the pain specialist, and 10 days after my last unproductive physical therapy session.

Since I won't be seeing the pain specialist for a while, I've decided to perform an experiment. I want to determine if massaging and stretching the muscles above the implants in every direction makes a difference. I will focus on the areas where my pectoral muscles attach to other muscles, such as under my left arm and under that clavicle. The manual manipulations might be more productive than aggressive stretches. Stretches seem to pull on painful nerves in the vicinity, and the combination has become a vicious cycle.

I am going to postpone Lyrica, at least for a few more days. If I obtain results I want to make sure they are from physical, not from chemical, interventions.

◈

Experiment Prompts a New Direction

April 4th

Extreme pectoral tension has been playing a *huge* role in my discomfort. The relief is most noticeable when I perform activities that pull or engage pectoral muscles, such as when I drive or recline, which would have been extremely painful a few weeks ago. Surprisingly, even the constant neck and chest tightness is also less intense.

Those results have managed to surprise, encourage, and disappoint me all at once. The relief is only temporary, the tightness is also present in other areas, and there is no way I can resolve this on my own. Trying to resolve extreme muscular tension barely addressed by constant stretches or muscle relaxants is the challenge here. Widespread muscular tension explains why my pain often subsides in varying degrees, and why it always recurs.

As I searched for suggestions, I came across *ART,* or *Advanced Release Technique*, a massage technique with certified practitioners throughout the United States. I am hopeful. My favorite article references a resource that suggests releasing muscles through trigger point compression and stretching, for those of us with myofascial dysfunctions [31,102]. And since I feel painful knots around my left shoulder, along the lateral aspects of my ribs, as well as under and behind both arms, the approach is worth trying. This is the best plan I've had in a long time.

◈

Unique Massages Provide Explanations

April 20th-22nd

I have gladly paid for five hours of additional pain to help relieve my pain. Of course I know it sounds crazy, and yes, it was probably desperate, but after experiencing a degree of nerve pain relief from Body Talk, I am willing to try complementary treatments. I am grateful for that desperate mindset. Without it, I might not have not taken the rehabilitative gamble I took. Had I not done that, I would not have won the rehabilitative lottery I feel I've won. No, I did not find a magic wand or an overnight recovery. What I found were answers and explanations, which I really needed, and those are helping to map out a new course of action. It is all so exciting that I am not even sure how to begin, though I suppose I can start where I left off after physical therapy.

Other than cervical compression confirmation, which is only mild to moderate in different areas, my neck and upper torso MRI results were negative. Those results left me feeling a little confused—I was starting to contemplate either a nerve block or trigger point injections. After the MRI report I discarded those ideas, even though they might have offered temporary relief. If the source of the pain is masked, I won't know how to resolve the problem that is causing it.

Through a ZIP code search at activerelease.com I found someone with a high level of training just a few miles from our home. My very capable ART practitioner agreed that extreme muscular tension is playing a significant role in my discomfort. He discovered abnormal knots at important muscle and tendon junctures around my left upper arm and shoulder.

He also found a lot of scar tissue. Interestingly, some of it is exactly where I've been feeling sharp pain just under my left arm. To avoid pressure on the implants, but still break up nearby scar tissue, he has me lie on the opposite side, which displaces them by gravity. The presence of so much scar tissue is surprising. Some rehabilitative literature suggests that scar tissue can be diminished with constant range-of-motion exercises and with gentle self-massages. I have been diligent with both, although my massages are not as deep as the ART technique demands. For lack of a better explanation, some of my muscles and tendons have been glued together. The unnatural fusion has kept them from working independently and could explain why physical therapy did not work. Scar tissue probably added pain and could have played a role with the capsular contracture.

Limited progress seems to be occurring with the few ART sessions I've had. My muscles feel a little less tense and are perhaps a little less painful. Most of all my instincts are telling me that I am moving in the right direction.

RELAY FOR LIFE EVENTS

May 1st

At this year's *Relay For Life* events, we were able to compare my year-to-year progress. Last year I was unable to complete the one lap designated for survivors. I was the most recent survivor at both fundraisers, although unfortunately, that was not the case this year.

Neil and Nicole experienced different emotions from time to time. Even though this year she was more composed, last year Nicole was very emotional and cried in her best friend's arms. I was not there, I was unable to stay. Neil did the opposite. He saved his tears for this year, and just when I thought he was unable to cry about my cancer. It happened while we were gazing at lit luminaries dedicated to family members who became cancer casualties, as well as my own. Knowing that my children have cried because of my cancer, on this and on other occasions, feels like daggers are piercing my heart. But since expressing their sadness is part of their healing, I am glad they were able to cry.

The luminaire ceremony was the most moving part. Even though the stadium lighting was turned off, the parameter remained lit by the hundreds of bright luminaries that surrounded the track. I was humbled when my 18-year-old son walked hand in hand with me in front of his peers. We observed the collective tribute to others who are, or were, related to the hundreds of teens who made the event a reality, and not surprisingly, many of those adolescents got tearful. Neil called the evening "my night" and promised to keep me company if I stayed, when I tried to leave early so he could spend time with his friends. How could I refuse?

Both Sandy and I accomplished our goals from last year. I wanted to wear a survivor T-shirt, and I was hoping to feel strong enough to walk several laps in honor of my survivorship. I accomplished both goals, although just barely with the first. I had to get a large T-shirt so that it would be loose around my chest and upper arms, and I had to be very liberal with my prescribed ointment. Sandy's goal was more challenging in a physical sense of the word. Last year he promised he would walk a lap at each relay with me on his shoulders. I tried to discourage him, but he would not be dissuaded. I finally agreed. He clarified he needed to do it for himself.

And so it was. He carried me on his shoulders for an entire lap at each relay, where I felt taller than I have ever felt before. As we observed other survivors, their families, and volunteers alike, it became clear that this gesture, which was Sandy's personal goal last year, was very touching for them as well.

I am glad we attended. The relays served as a progress reminder. We had a chance to get in touch with our emotions, and I got to speak with several breast cancer survivors.

⚜

Scar Tissue

May 5th

When pressed, scar tissue has a very specific sensation. It feels as though there is a long fingernail being dug deep into the skin. Having deep scar tissue broken up by ART can be painful and it might take several sessions, and yet, I go willingly. Compared to the physical therapy massages, the pain reprieves are longer.

Knowing how scar tissue feels has allowed me to identify similar sensations. I found scar tissue under both *areolar circumferences* (the nipple and the surrounding dark skin), between the implants, and under both scars. Logic dictates that ART massages might not be appropriate directly on the incisions or over the implants, which is why I've been performing those massages. Last week my plastic surgeon confirmed my suspicion. With nipple-sparing mastectomies, the areolar areas tend to develop more scar tissue.

I also learned that those of us who choose a mastectomy develop most of our scar tissue in the first year. Two layers of scar tissue try to form; the upper layer of the pectoral muscles might wind up with scar tissue from the skin, which is just above, *and* from the implants, which are positioned just underneath. That can be problematic. The pectoral muscles are involved in most upper-body movements. My plastic surgeon does not believe creams can break up scar tissue. That is logical, since much of it forms *under* the skin.

All of this information explains why my chest-pulling sensations continue to diminish. The added comfort makes sense. If scar tissue has been attached to skin, tendons, or muscles, their ability to flex and/or stretch has been limited.

Preventing scar tissue is an ongoing battle and some of us are more prone. I seem to have a higher predisposition. My family history and my darker pigmentation could have contributed. My plastic surgeon pointed out that many doctors do not believe massages can make a difference in scar tissue management, although based on what I have been able to accomplish, in such a short period of time, I believe massages can help some of us.

⚜

MUSCULAR IMBALANCE PROGRESSION

May 7th-10th

Understanding the *sequence* of events that led to my present deficits might be the only way to come up with an effective plan. Tracking the muscular imbalance progression was not as hard as I thought it would be, thanks to this journal, to the knowledge I gained in physical therapy, and from my recent research.

In retrospect, the biggest loss of movement and sensation were to my upper arms, axillae, and into my back for a few inches at that same level. The journal reminded me that initially my arms were unable to move in any direction, other than in a straight up-and-down motion, and at no more than a 90-degree angle. I also remembered that even though my right arm healed sequentially, the difficulties to my left arm progressed.

Those same muscles, which typically rely on the *posterior* branch of the *axillary nerve,* are still the weakest, and they are just starting to regain sensation. By name my left *posterior deltoid muscle,* located in the back of the arm, might have been a casualty. Since both depend on the same nerve branch, and both are needed to support and rotate that shoulder and scapula, my left *teres minor* and *infraspinatus* muscles might have also been affected. Such nerve disruptions, and then muscular imbalances, would explain my difficulties writing, pushing, pressing, rotating, lifting, and how heavy my left arm has felt. Weakness and lost muscle mass to the front of my left arm followed over time. It was not present originally, but it is now.

Sometime after that, the forward displacement of my left shoulder and scapula occurred. The combination of weak pectoral muscles, weak shoulder muscles, and weak upper-back muscles, were unable to hold them in place. In fact, for a time my left shoulder remained rolled forward when I lay down. Scar tissue, leaning forward in a protective manner to diminish pain, and the weight of the left implant, added to the left shoulder and scapula displacements.

The multiple dysfunctions could explain why my trapezius muscle, which diamonds from the base of the skull, fans out to both shoulders, and then makes its final attachment in the middle of the spine, eventually got so tight. That muscle was trying to help, but it caused more muscular imbalances and tension. Trapezius tightness can explain several familiar symptoms: mid-back pain, shoulder pain, neck pain, as well as headaches [40].

I am finally prepared to accept long-term limitations. There are too many issues to ignore that possibility. Accepting slow progress is better than frustration;

a defeated mindset might discourage new attempts. But not yet, not now, it is too soon to give up trying. I am still making progress.

❦

RUDIMENTARY REHABILITATIVE PLAN

May 20th

Now that I have a better understanding of my abnormal muscular compensations, and since a lot of my scar tissue has been addressed, I am trying to come up with a sequential strengthening plan.

Because they appear to be the weakest, it might be important to find movements that allow the muscles in the back of my left arm and shoulder to move without pain. Although such motion needs to be very limited, otherwise the muscles between my left shoulder and neck engage. So far, the one motion that does not perpetuate the cycle is the constant motion from a brisk walk. And since walking is so easy, gentle, and effective, I do it for at least two hours a week, although in short intervals. It is still tiring. I am again able to walk on a regular basis. The lymphedema symptoms have completely subsided.

To start strengthening the muscles in the back of my left arm, I am performing posterior butterfly exercises daily; although, it is important to press down between my left shoulder and neck and limit the angle to 30 degrees away from my torso, otherwise the wrong muscles tighten. I have been gradually increasing the repetitions and the amount of weight. After slowly progressing at half-pound increments, I am now able to lift one and one-half pounds without neck and shoulder pain. That might seem slow, but it has taken a month to achieve, and it is a lot more than I could do in physical therapy.

The other important goal is to relax the tight trapezius muscle. Keeping in mind the location and the sheer size of that muscle, I have been placing each hand on the opposite shoulder blade. Then with my head tucked in as far forward as I can, I gradually lower my torso as far as possible. Next I bring my shoulder blades back, and do several shoulder and neck rotations. In physical therapy I learned that to help them relax, muscles need to be pulled together and stretched in the opposite direction.

Part of the plan should include efforts that help my left shoulder and scapula return to their intended locations. Standing and sitting with my back straight and with both shoulders rolled back seem to be helping. My six-week physical therapist taught me several exercises to ease these problems. To roll my shoulder blades back in an exaggerated fashion, and to lie on an exercise roll, as it supports my head and spine. I also stand with my arms resting at my sides, and then elevate them slowly and simultaneously until they meet above my head. That seemingly simple motion, also learned in physical therapy, is meant to help my shoulders regain their lost symmetry. Aside from those, I am focusing on very gentle, controlled movements in every direction.

To make sure I am moving in perfect symmetry, I try to perform most exercises in front of a mirror. The mirror visual is a perfect opportunity to remind my body that it can again move painlessly, symmetrically, and with strength. I try to *feel* and *visualize* the symmetry so that I can duplicate it by feel alone for the rest of the day.

Strengthening efforts also require proper posture. I need to perform the described exercise while standing perfectly straight. Bending engages the wrong muscles and keeps the intended ones from moving. During my walks and throughout the day, I make sure my abdominal muscles are tucked in, and that both shoulders are equally rolled back.

I've learned a lot by paying attention. From trying to determine if specific movements, angle of lifting, or positioning cause pain, I've realized that my arms should not support my torso. I also have to stay away from bands, or any type of heavy lifting. All of them set me back for days. Physical therapy is not possible, not now. My plan was to return when I could perform the prescribed exercises consecutively and with less pain, but my tolerance is still limited to just two to three minutes at a time. Besides, most of the physical therapy exercises were at shoulder level, and at that angle the pain is intense and immediate.

Ultimately, I want to lower the need for the wrong muscles to overwork, encourage my weaker ones to return to their proper roles, and diminish all of the pain. Since my muscular tension will probably persist (or increase) as I try to reverse these dysfunctional patterns, I will carry on with professional massages. Above all, I will proceed at a gradual and tolerable pace that keeps me moving forward. My body has spoken loud and clear: it will not be rushed.

DIMINISHED PAIN

May 24th

I sought ART massages to diminish chest and shoulder tightness, which is unquestionably being achieved, though quite unexpectedly much of my residual nerve sensitivity has improved, to a degree that seemed unattainable.

The process has been trial and error. When one of the massages was performed below my left axilla, nerve sensitivity in that area increased for several days. The risk paid off. A nerve must have been entrapped by scar tissue. Now, three weeks later, the area feels better than it did before this episode. The experience taught me that Lyrica can lower nerve sensitivity, and yet I am glad I postponed it. Lyrica at an earlier stage might have kept me from pursuing ART massages, and that would have been a mistake. I've stopped Lyrica. It too made me feel depressed.

From a wardrobe perspective, my improved level of comfort is as welcome as it is unexpected. I can finally wear slightly fitted sleeves in proximity to the previously untouchable areas in the back of my arms. I started to *shop* in my own closet. Every single new shirt is now worn with the proper appreciation for that typically mundane activity. Many shirts still get uncomfortable after a couple of hours if my muscles are sore *and* tight. The combination seems to reawaken nerve sensitivity, though that is happening to a lesser extent and with less frequency. In addition to my few spaghetti-strap shirts, my slightly more comfortable wardrobe now consists of one robe, two thin ¾-sleeved jackets, two large-sleeved shirts, and one closed black sweater I actually like. On two occasions I wore one of my big soft-sleeved shirts for the entire day! I can once again wear cotton. Cotton used to hurt and that had become a dilemma. My hot flashes needed cotton, while my sensitive nerves could only tolerate polyester.

Getting to know which muscles need to be released by combining massages and stretches has been important, especially if the location is considered a *trigger point*. Now that most of my scar tissue has been addressed, some of those trigger points seem to respond to deep-tissue massages. Others are aggravated by them, and yet others feel better with massages around the discomfort. I started massaging sore muscles if I can reach them, not only because the discomfort has lessened and the massages are draining our budget, only I can work on the uncomfortable locations daily. From self-massages I've learned that some areas feel tender to the touch, long before they started hurting. Even though the *back* of my neck is what hurts, the pain is worsened by tight tendons and muscles in the *front* of my neck. If I intervene early I can minimize, or delay, the eventual discomfort.

Since I can again lie on my stomach, I've returned to my pre-mastectomy massage therapist every other week. Those gentler massages should relieve tightness in weak muscles; those muscles now feel like they used to feel when I had a good workout prior to my double mastectomy. The difference is that this soreness persists for days at a time and builds up incrementally if it is not massaged, even though I still stretch constantly, although I will probably need to do that for the rest of my life.

⌘

AN ATYPICAL MUSCULAR PAIN THEORY

June 12th

Approximately three weeks ago I had a new concerning experience. I did not record it at the time. It did not seem related to my breast cancer complications, but it might be related after all.

For a time exercising became far more challenging. I was getting lightheaded, I got a strong headache, and I always felt very tired afterwards. I persevered, even though my stamina was decreasing and I was doing less and less. I have not forgotten my promise to the medical oncologist: I would exercise regularly and vigorously to help prevent a recurrence. The basic things had been ruled out. My blood sugar, iron, and other lab work appeared normal, and I was eating well. My pulse was regular, strong, not abnormally fast, and I was not short of breath. I assumed I was just getting old and tired. Then on one particular day I developed a much stronger headache, even though I had only walked a mile that felt more like ten.

On the way home I checked my blood pressure at the grocery store and it was very elevated, particularly my *diastolic* pressure, the lower number. In light of the double mastectomy, and to diminish compression to my upper arms, I bought a wrist blood pressure cuff. I've been checking my blood pressure on the right wrist. That side had fewer lymph nodes removed and no swelling episodes.

Right before cancer treatment I started hypothyroidism medicine, which is why I was trying to determine whether I needed a cardiologist or an endocrinologist. When I began to explore a possible connection between hypothyroidism and blood pressure abnormalities, I understood that even though there are other culprits, thyroid hormone deficiencies can cause hypertension [105,150,165]. The agent that might be deficient is *nitric oxide,* and L-Arginine, an over-the-counter amino acid, is a nitric oxide *precursor*. I checked with my primary doctor to make sure the supplement was safe to try until the endocrinology appointment four weeks later. Then I worked at finding the lowest dose to ease my symptoms, except I found much more.

By decreasing my overall muscular tension, L-Arginine has serendipitously improved my rehabilitation. The added comfort extends beyond my upper-torso— *all* of the muscles throughout my body feel more at ease. Even aches to my hips and back, which I thought had become my constant companions, are less noticeable. Some days they are downright absent. I am not as tired, I comfortably added more weight, and I increased the frequency of my left arm-strengthening efforts.

I've since learned that stress factors, such as major surgeries, can aggravate hypothyroidism. Such a scenario could have interfered with my muscular healing after all of the surgeries, during the implant migration, or at least with the frozen shoulder. My constant mobility, even through pain, should have prevented that complication. I am very excited about all of this, having an explanation could mean finding a solution. I look forward to an in-depth discussion with an endocrinologist.

The hypothyroidism-pain connection seems important. Some breast cancer experts have written about the need to identify women who are at risk for long-term pain so they can be monitored. I suddenly have a profile for mine: personal and family history of muscular pain, a propensity to scar tissue (from family history and from ethnicity), nerve damage from surgery, hypothyroidism, and asthma. What a perfect pain storm.

⅏

NERVE HEALING STAGES

June 15th

My inability to tolerate medicines for pain has allowed me to feel each nerve healing stage. The sensations have been unpredictable, but the progression could be over soon. The odd sensations feel more topical, are less frequent, and even their intensity has dramatically diminished.

The worst and longest stage was from late September until mid-spring—the allodynia period. During those months I could not get comfortable, dressed or undressed. I've since read that some women are able to feel comfortable without clothes during that stage. I was not that lucky. My pectoral muscles hurt with the weight of the implants. I began to wonder if I had made a mistake with the reconstruction. These days I only need support during the day, but for months it was necessary at night. It is hard to believe these implants were in my chest wall last fall.

Progress is slowly occurring, but some things are still far from normal. Aluminum deodorants still produce immediate discomfort when applied to my left axilla, although that axilla has not been perspiring. Sandy believes the lack of perspiration, along with the numbness in the area, can be blamed on nerve damage. The skin that covers the back of my left upper arm and neck actually hurts when I am in a cold room or standing under a fan. If I had been able to wear sleeves, as I now can, this stage would have been preferable in the winter. Instead, it is happening in the middle of a Florida June, filled with fans and air conditioning. This stage is easier to manage—I am just hoping it is the last.

Even though the progression was painful, there is one positive outcome from my nerve regeneration. Aside from both areolar complexes, and a quarter of my right reconstructed side, I regained my chest sensation. Was the discomfort worthwhile? I don't know. What I do know is that the lack of sensation made the skin on my chest feel very, very, strange.

ΞΒΘ

ENDOCRINOLOGIST VALIDATES MUSCULAR PAIN THEORY

June 25th

It has been confirmed. Strictly by coincidence I found an important pain-puzzle piece. Let me explain. All of my symptoms, including my muscular pain, indicate that my *TSH level* (the main laboratory value used to determine thyroid function) needs to be much lower. It might need to be as low as one or close to zero, instead of where it presently is at the high end of normal on the lab report. Aside from validating a possible connection between hypothyroidism and my ongoing pain, the endocrinologist stated that as long as my blood pressure was not getting too low, L-Arginine can be used to increase my exercise tolerance. And since the supplement helped to lower my blood pressure, I do not need to consult a cardiologist.

Even so, just to be on the safe side, I am no longer using L-Arginine. Research taught me that it might worsen asthma symptoms, and the most detailed book I found points to the possibility of increased cancer cell proliferation through indirect means [47]. Some of the clinical studies were inconclusive, but others pointed to a negative, vague connection, a suspicion that was the conclusion of a separate study [45]. The negative effects could be the result of high doses, and I do miss the sense of well-being from the supplement, but adequate thyroid medicine should provide the same benefits. My rehabilitation continues to progress at a faster pace than before this episode, but adjusting to a new dose and type of thyroid medicine is exhausting.

~~~

Why Did I Get Cancer? Did Endocrine Issues Contribute?

July 20th-22nd

Cancer survivorship is about so much more than just being alive. All of us survivors eventually wonder *why did I get cancer? How can I help prevent a recurrence?* Although for some of us, the answers are not that clear.

Yes, I know what the experts recommend: exercise, eat a low-fat diet, have a low body mass index, and don't smoke or drink in excess. But what if I had been doing all of those things and I still got cancer? Have I gone organic? Not much really, somehow that does not seem like my answer. I am no longer using plastic in the microwave, I am eating less red meat, I use fewer artificial sweeteners, and I drink less bottled water. Doing all of that is fulfilling the need to do something, but I don't think I am preventing a recurrence.

And yet, there is one loose string that needs tying, a possibility that has recently become a probable factor. I want to let go of *the* questions, even though this is probably the result of overthinking and reading too much. It has been eight weeks since I used L-Arginine for a month, and another month since I started the new thyroid medicine. My blood pressure is no longer elevated, and the lightening of muscular aches throughout my body continues to be nothing short of miraculous.

That is not all. The daily headaches and the numerous hot flashes that I've had for years are less frequent and intense. The last improvement is particularly welcome. Since I could not take supplements or hormones to lessen the hot flashes, they were a constant cancer reminder. I found some consolation in knowing they could have been worse with aromatase inhibitors, which I barely avoided. Other than information on how the thyroid gland plays a role in temperature regulation [89], I've found no explanation for the improvement. But if my blood vessels are getting what they need, then that too might be lowering hot flashes. My hot flashes feel vascular. They worsen when I lie down or turn in bed.

All of this relief has made me wonder if I had thyroid disease, long before it was diagnosed. In my early 40s I began to struggle with various symptoms that are also improving. I suffered with continued tiredness, I had difficulty concentrating, I had muscular aches, I dealt with recurrent depression, and I developed high cholesterol. The last two symptoms are also risk factors for heart disease—where I was recently heading. The antidepressants and synthetic hormones I was prescribed for years worked poorly, perhaps they were not what I needed; hypothyroidism symptoms can be similar to those of menopause or perimenopause [138,145]. In *The Wisdom of Menopause,* Dr. Christiane Northrup, M.D., mentions that a quarter of women develop hypothyroidism during or close to perimenopause, and that the problem can be worsened by supplemental estrogen [127].

Those hormones might have played a role in the hiding of my breast cancer. One theory is that my prescribed combination of estrogen and progesterone (or progestin), might slow the natural decrease of dense tissue that typically occurs with aging [164].

Vitamin D is not as well absorbed with poor thyroid function. Vitamin D was the one vitamin my medical oncologist recommended and the one that was typically low in my blood work, even though I took a supplement and frequently spent time outdoors.

I didn't just find a theory for the why did I get cancer question, I found something that can help address my cancer recurrence concerns. To lower breast cancer (and heart disease) risk factors, I will try to keep my endocrine system in balance.

~❧~

MEDICAL APPOINTMENTS & FEAR OF RECURRENCES

August 5th

These days I dread the history and physical pages at routine doctor's appointments. I do not like to include my breast cancer diagnosis, the dual mastectomy, and the neuromuscular pain. Yes, I know I should include them. Honestly, I always have. But do the dentist, the allergist, and the eye doctor need to know so much? Would it really break some medical record ethics code if I were to exclude those details and only disclosed the ones that are important to each setting? Besides, the information can lead to an uncomfortable discussion, such as how I was diagnosed, which sometimes leaves the female health care providers concerned.

I am no longer undergoing cancer treatment, and yet every practitioner feels the need to make sure cancer is not present in the body part of their expertise.

It all started in the fall after my gynecological appointment, when postmenopausal bleeding caused the uterine cancer scare. That episode was followed by less-eventful cancer screenings at the dentist's, and the ophthalmologist's offices. I also had X-rays at the pain specialist's consultation, and now I wonder if he too was looking for cancer. Recently my endocrinologist ordered a thyroid ultrasound, but I did not bother to ask why.

Screenings have been considered necessary, although perhaps because of the testing I underwent I am no longer interested in pursuing further screenings to rule anything in, or to rule anything out. Every resource indicates that a metastatic recurrence would make itself clear. The long-term prognosis appears to be the same either way.

It is impossible to get away from the idea of a cancer recurrence. I think of that possibility every time I massage my scars. A *local* recurrence is sometimes visible or palpable, and often noted along incision lines. This type of recurrence can be successfully treated if it is caught in time, although the same cannot be said of a distant one. Regardless of where it is found, it is metastatic. Finding something unusual on my chest would be easy. There is only a thin layer of muscle between the implants and my skin, and the implant softness would make it easy to find irregularities. Therefore, keeping the area as scar-free as possible is a motivation from the recurrence-detection perspective, as well as from the obvious cosmetic and comfort incentives.

I am very vigilant. I have memorized, and will continue monitoring, the look and sensation of every palpable bump. No irregularity on my chest, neck, or axillae would go unnoticed. I frequently inspect all of those areas, I just try not to do it in fear. I try to do it with a sense of love. That part of my body has suffered enough and does not need my disdain. I learned this concept from Dr. Susan Northrup, M.D. With the exclusion of women with a new breast cancer diagnosis, we should perform caring massages to get in touch with ourselves, not militant, fearful breast exams [127].

Perhaps as time goes by my medical appointments will settle into a new normal that is not so abnormal.

⚬⚬⚬

REHABILITATIVE SETBACK

August 11th

I've been trying to gradually increase my strength, but progress is slow. It took over six weeks to increase left arm weight bearing from two to five pounds, and even that seems too fast. The left arm is still weaker than the right. I will start bilateral exercises when my strength feels equal. That could happen soon; the difference is narrowing. The real breakthrough, if that day ever comes, will be when I can lift 10 pounds with combined arm effort; most upper-body machines at the gym start at that level. The ability to use some of that equipment would open up a new world of exercise options.

I am getting way ahead of myself. I need to somehow ease the tension between my left shoulder and neck, as well as the pain between my upper-neck vertebrae. Both have worsened. Instead of helping, strengthening efforts are once again aggravating them. Physical therapy for a third time might be worth a try. If I can at least gain a little strength, the effort will be worth the hassle.

At least I found validation. My neck, arm, and shoulder problems are known breast cancer treatment side effects [153]. The knowledge that others are in pain does not provide consolation. It is just nice to have justification for these issues, which would otherwise seem unrelated.

～

LIMITED THIRD PHYSICAL THERAPY EXPERIENCE

September 8th-10th

Even though this time I looked for a senior physical therapist who regularly works with breast cancer patients, my last physical therapy attempt was both helpful and disappointing.

At our first meeting she seemed to understand why my previous experiences were unproductive. I explained that I took a step back when I progressed to lifting 5 pounds, even though I've continued with regular massages, and I still limit lateral and posterior left arm strengthening movements to 30 degrees away from my torso. I told her that my left shoulder was depressed for a while, but that these days it again looks higher than the right. I clarified that the muscles between my left shoulder and neck are again shortened, feel tight, and are just as sore as they were a few months ago. On that note she gave me a good tip. Instead of just rolling my left shoulder back to help it reposition, I should also be pressing it *down*.

How could I have missed something so simple and obvious? My left shoulder is not as rolled forward, which is progress, but since I've not been pressing it down that shoulder assumed a higher position, and several neck muscles retightened.

She gave me suggestions for working at the computer, an activity that is still very uncomfortable. I need to sit with my back straight and with both shoulders rolled back and pressed down. To keep upper arms and shoulders from moving, both wrists should remain on the surface of the computer, and the height of the computer needs to be at elbow level. In other words, motion should only be *below* the elbows. To limit neck bending, and the ensuing neck discomfort, I have been raising the back of the laptop by several inches.

As far as recommended exercise, none were new. We specifically discussed the one where I move my arms forward by approximately 45 degrees, then *very* slowly bring them up to shoulder level while keeping them extended. The goal is to keep both shoulders equally leveled. That exercise (best performed in front of a mirror) is supposed to help isolate and retrain shoulder muscles, except my left shoulder tends to rise more than the right, particularly if I move too fast. I will now need to perform that exercise with my shoulder blades not only rolled back, but also pressed down. We reviewed two other familiar exercises. The one where I roll my shoulders back as far as I can and hold for a few seconds, and the slow side-to-side neck stretches while pressing down on the opposite shoulder.

It was suggested I refrain from using heavy weights and again train with one pound. That makes sense, except I'm not sure how to actually strengthen my arms without using more weight. And if the muscles on my left arm are not strong, the vicious cycle will be perpetuated.

I went to the second appointment two weeks later, I am progressing that slowly. The therapist agreed, even though she was hoping I schedule more frequent sessions. I explained that I need time to make sure the new recommendations are not worsening the problem. She understood. In fact, she added it might take another year to regain some strength. Unfortunately my snail's pace progress is more than day-to-day inconvenience, and well beyond personal frustration. Unless progress can be documented from week to week, my insurance company will not pay for the therapy, and each referral is only good for one month. She suggested I get a new referral each time I need help, except that seems cumbersome and unrealistic.

The option seemed worth contemplating, at least until she implied that I should begin to acknowledge my inability to improve. I am neither prepared to accept, nor contemplate, such a concept. Since the therapist seems so knowledgeable I might consider going back. On the other hand, it might be hard to progress with someone who starts with a defeated attitude.

This is concerning. What do others who have to work for a living do? Since repetitive arm movement aggravates all of the pain, I would be unable to perform any job that requires constant motion, and that would probably be most jobs. She suggested that as soon as that happens I should stop, stretch, ice, and rest. Those interventions are helpful, but not realistic when I am driving, cooking, or grocery shopping. They are also incapable of reversing the problem. I believe I will eventually figure this out, even if I stumble a few times, but professional guidance would have been nice.

⤰

CANCER TRAVEL OUTLOOK

October 2nd

We have completed our third out-of-state trip. That's a lot of traveling for us, except this year we had good excuses. We had two out-of-state weddings, including Andrew's. Those trips were not only wonderful, they proved that I am now seeing life from a different perspective.

Due to the limited lifting and straining, and because I took a rehabilitative break, a nearly comfortable vacation with my family felt like a dream come true. That was unexpected. I thought I would no longer experience traveling comfort. I was less uncomfortable in the car for hours at a time, although I still needed an arsenal of strategically placed pillows to support my arms and upper back. I could not move any of the large suitcases, but I did push my small carry-on for brief intervals. All of those were milestones, but the *most* luxurious thing was the ability to wear long sleeves, T-shirts, and jackets all week, even though they still had to be large and soft.

Going to unique places and spending time with family have become particularly enjoyable, and cancer is responsible for the new outlook. I was never someone who enjoyed outdoor destinations, but that too has changed. As we were driving through California's Big Sur, admiring the majestic redwood trees in Northern California, seeing the imposing mountains in Montana, and spending two days in Yellowstone National Park, I felt like I was at holy places, not just visiting beautiful outdoor locations. The physical challenges that some of the visitors were experiencing at Yellowstone National Park, point to the possibility of it being a favorite bucket-list destination, and I can certainly understand why.

When I was at the Metropolitan Museum, and the Museum of Modern Art in New York City, I also had unexpected experiences. As I examined my favorite Van Gogh and Monet paintings, I felt tears on my cheeks. I took in their sheer beauty, perhaps for the very first time. That was atypical. When it comes to display of emotions, I'm usually very private.

I have always been the designated vacation and financial planner, but prior to cancer I never felt comfortable splurging on our vacations. Paying down our house, getting rid of a car payment, funding a savings account, or completing a home-improvement project took priority over our travel needs. Those priorities will no longer apply. Upgrading to a nicer room, staying a few extra days, and having dinner at the nicer restaurant feels like we are living! I've not changed my mind. Being responsible is essential, though suddenly, so is enjoying life a little more. Now I wonder, what is the point of saving money if something happens and we never got to enjoy it? Increased spending after cancer is not atypical—it has been labeled cancer spending.

At the family weddings I was able to dance and delight at having our children together looking healthy and happy. Seeing how in love Andrew and Lauren are filled my heart with joy. Those are the kind of days that give life a heightened meaning. They make the struggles of a health crisis worthwhile, although I probably saw it that way more than others did at those joyful gatherings, filled with so many dear friends and family members.

Spending time alone with Sandy and rediscovering each other away from work, routine, stress, health issues, and family responsibilities was overdue. We have been doing a lot of talking, as recommended, but since it was such a healing experience, what we really needed was to stop talking and start enjoying things together again.

As wonderful as those experiences were, we cannot afford endless traveling and we cannot avoid day-to-day responsibilities. At home, routine activities now seem more monotonous and time consuming. During those times my mind wanders towards future ambivalences. Cancer and its future uncertainties have moved into our home, into our minds, and into our lives. The new challenge is to find joy in the routine and continue the momentum generated by those trips. Being part of that routine has been a privilege, I should never take that for granted. Maybe what I need to do is stop panicking into the future, find the ordinary more extraordinary, and then do it as frequently as possible.

COMPLEMENTARY CANCER CARE CONFERENCE

October 10th

Recently Tatiana and I attended the annual conference for gynecological and for breast cancer survivors, hosted by Moffit Cancer Center. Being in a room with hundreds of other women who have been touched by cancer was incredible. Some of them are still undergoing treatment, but they were still poised and beautiful.

Discussing seemingly taboo subjects was easy and informative. Some women spoke about their experiences with asymmetry and infections. One survivor explained why she turned away anti-estrogen therapy; in her case as in mine, the risks outweighed the benefits. Other women openly verbalized their discomfort about the inappropriate jokes and comments some people make about our reconstructed bodies. A psychologist suggested we verbalize our discomfort on the spot, while keeping in mind that those comments are made by people who don't know what else to say.

Several specialists provided important information. I heard a prominent plastic surgeon explain how he only performs tissue-graft reconstructions on tissue that has received radiation. In his view, elasticity for implant reconstructions is lost with radiation. He mentioned in passing that nerve damage and muscular trauma are risks from *any* surgery. At that moment I wondered how many others found the statement to be as much a part of their experience as I did. I joyfully learned from a nutritionist that tofu and soybeans can be eaten in cautious moderation, even by those of us with estrogen-receptor positive cancers (ER+). I was glad. I have been avoiding and missing them in my diet. One panelist spoke about how normal it is to fear a recurrence. It was explained that we need to learn to live with the uncertainty without letting it take over our lives. She emphasized that sometimes our family members do not understand those concerns, which is why connecting with other survivors in some fashion is so important on an ongoing basis.

The actual focus of the conference was even more interesting. The emphasis was on an *integrative* medical approach to ease treatment stress and undesirable long-term effects. The idea is to take into consideration mental and spiritual needs, while merging traditional cancer therapies with *complementary* methods. By definition complementary treatments do *not* interfere with traditional medicine. I also learned that many major cancer centers offer massage therapy, meditation, art therapy, journaling, and visualization guidance. One of the speakers was a medical doctor who is also trained in the art of acupuncture. She explained that just like her, many other physicians are graduating from medical school with the same training.

We learned that it would be a mistake to turn to *alternative* therapies, which are substitutes for traditional approaches, such as chemotherapy. They also cautioned against taking supplements that may interfere with cancer treatments. Those mistakes can be avoided by researching, and by checking with our primary doctors and our oncologists. As I listened to all of those experts, I felt that many of my approaches were validated. I've used, and continue to use, many of those complementary therapies to regain a sense of well-being.

⊗⊘◎

BREAST CANCER AWARENESS MONTH

October 17th

After the United States Preventive Services Task Force's (USPSTF) recommendations, and without the emphasis on early and frequent breast cancer screenings, this Breast Cancer Awareness Month is unrecognizable. Last October there were many stories in the newspaper and on the internet from women who benefitted from some type of early screening. I was hoping those voices would again make themselves heard, louder than ever. But it did not happen. Most of those voices were silent this year.

How will the new recommendations affect women who are not aware of their risk? The overwhelming majority of women diagnosed with breast cancer do not have a genetic predisposition, a first-degree relative with breast cancer, or even a second-degree relative with the disease [112]. Will annual mammograms for most women under the age of 50 really stop? Is it possible that self-exams will no longer be the norm? If insurance companies stop covering annual mammograms, will more women receive a late-stages diagnosis? Can diminished awareness limit fundraising contributions, and therefore research?

Some have suggested that annual breast cancer screenings are not cost effective. Strictly from a financial perspective, shouldn't the cost of a late diagnosis also be considered? An advanced diagnosis increases the need for chemotherapy, the likelihood of complications, and can result in additional surgeries. More women would require premature end-of-life care, which would also add to the cost.

There are plenty of studies to support both sides of the mammogram debate though in my situation, the new guidelines made me glad that my history of breast cancer will allow Nicole to undergo frequent breast cancer screenings without much opposition.

All of this was on my mind at a follow-up appointment. Two-thirds of the patients in the waiting area had something else in common with me, other than their probable breast cancer: they seemed to be under the age of 50.

❧

LACK OF ANSWERS & COMPLEMENTARY APPROACHES

November 19th

I have not written about my physical discomforts for over two months—or about anything else for an entire month. I was beginning to feel that even my journal was tired of my unresolved issues and my continued setbacks, but I am finally ready to write again.

Looking at the calendar I am reminded of my last endocrinologist appointment. I was forced to report that I was again very tired, perhaps even more so than I was a couple of months ago. I shared that I often felt lightheaded when I got up from a sitting or a lying down position. I explained that I could not work out, even though my muscles were less sore and my blood pressure was no longer elevated—it was getting very low. My endocrinologist did not believe an endocrine imbalance was to blame, but I felt certain that was the culprit.

Not long after that consultation I felt even more out of sorts. It took me a while to figure out that it was at least in part due to a mislabeled batch of thyroid medicine, although at that point I had been taking it for six weeks. The identification helped, but it did not take away all of the concerning symptoms. I reported my unusual symptoms to the on call endocrinology nurse. She did not believe they were endocrine in nature. I had to look for answers elsewhere.

The situation did not seem related to my breast cancer experience, but then I was proven wrong. When the thyroid replacement dosage was lowered, due to the sense of overmedication and the unknown mislabeling, my upper-torso pain increased dramatically. Hypothyroidism has been prolonging my muscular pain.

Aside from that, and perhaps because of it, I lost rehabilitative ground. As I explained in a previous entry, the muscles between my left shoulder and neck retightened, and I had to curtail my strengthening efforts. And even though prior to this episode I had been making progress with the pain between my neck vertebrae, it did not take long for that to increase—again. I started to consider a chiropractor.

The cervical compression needs addressing, but such progress would be unsustainable. The compression cannot resolve unless the muscular tension is properly addressed.

I must admit that for a few weeks I found the sum of my setbacks, my inability to find answers, and my lack of progress very depressing. I began to wonder if being in constant pain, sensing so much fatigue, experiencing mental fogginess, and feeling so out of sorts was really going to be the permanent state of affairs. Giving up, rather than searching for the impossible, crossed my mind. Then the mislabeling was identified, the pharmaceutical was substituted, and my muscles began to relax. Three weeks later I am able to view the world from a slightly better perspective. The pain is not gone, it is just more manageable. I am still very tired, but not like I was for several weeks.

After contemplating the situation from different perspectives, my integrative doctor and I decided to address the situation as a type of *adrenal insufficiency*. We considered this possibility because I have so many predisposing factors, including extreme, prolonged pain; a recent thyroid upheaval; and ongoing stress. With an advanced adrenal insufficiency very low cortisol levels might make functioning very difficult, although he explained that the condition is hard to diagnose without an invasive test.

The plan to address the condition was started on the third week of October. It calls for more rest, increased meditations, and any effort capable of lowering stress. Frequent meals to maximize my energy, specific food avoidances and inclusions, as well as carefully chosen adrenal supplements are part of the plan. I am not working out other than taking short walks, performing light yoga exercises, and continuing my frequent stretches. Acupuncture seemed worth trying. It has no side effects and it might help with the pain and the energy issues. This time I looked for a highly trained practitioner in a reputable medical establishment. I found such a person. After just three sessions I have a little more energy for day-to-day activities. My new acupuncturist agrees with the physician/acupuncturist from the Moffit Cancer Center conference: if acupuncture is going to be effective, results should be seen within three to five sessions.

Yet another comment from that conference is reassuring. One specialist pointed out that full recovery can take as long, or longer, as it took for the actual illness or treatment to run its course. I don't know if the reference applies, or if my ongoing difficulties would be considered part of the initial problem, I am just choosing to believe both apply for the sake of sanity.

New Muscular Imbalance

November 22nd-24th

Comparing chiropractic services was beneficial, even though I am not yet working with a chiropractor. I learned that some of those offices have massage therapists familiar with chronic muscular dysfunctions. Yes, I will admit it—my pain syndrome is considered *chronic*. I am just not prepared to accept the label also means *permanent*, not at this level of discomfort.

If nerves can take up to two years to regenerate, then the muscles affected might take just as long or longer to regain their balance. Then the involved muscles need to be strengthened, stretched, and massaged properly, all of which also takes a while. The process through which my nerves have healed was described by one chiropractor: those nerves have "sprouted." In other words, they have created alternative branches. Such a scenario would explain why I now have more strength and sensation than I did a year and a half ago.

After a lot of inquiring, I decided to work with a massage therapist from one of those practices, even though they do not take our insurance. But she came as highly regarded, as I am getting desperate. After a few massages, and based on how I feel, I am convinced she was an amazing find. I should know. She is the sixth massage therapist I've tried over the past eight months. I'm glad I did not give up looking. Her massages are very effective. She combines different techniques, but with an emphasis on trigger point release.

My new massage therapist pointed out what I should already know. Multiple muscles are needed for every movement, and since muscular pain can be *referred* (felt in other areas), surrounding muscles also need to be massaged. In other words, I've been putting too much emphasis on relaxing painful neck and shoulder muscles. To remedy my omission, her massages are covering my entire back, shoulders, arms, neck, and lateral muscles on both sides of my torso.

The new massages are timely. My *right* scapula is starting to *wing*, or protrude, in an unnatural manner. This new muscular dysfunction can be blamed on how my right arm has been doing more than its share of lifting and pulling for a while. Interestingly, I have no pain on that side, although the tendons on the right side of my neck (front and back) are tight and painful when I massage them. The same applies to the muscles inside the natural depression just off my right clavicle (a neck muscle trigger point).

I am not worried. In fact, I am hopeful. I know exactly how to keep the problem from progressing and how to reverse it, thanks to what I learned in physical therapy, and to what I've tried and read over the past several months. To encourage bilateral strength and symmetry, I need to perform the same exercises I've been attempting but on both sides. Since it could do so much more, I had wrongly assumed that my right side did not need attention. Bilateral strengthening is finally appropriate. Though not yet equal, my strength feels similar. Besides, my right side cannot heal without an intermittent break. After so many difficulties, my goal is to become ambidextrous.

Paying for so many massages and acupuncture treatments without remorse is atypical of me. It proves that pain and lack of answers tend to loosen the wallet. Desperate times can prompt unconventional measures.

∼∽∾

PROGRESS!

December 20th-26th

Even though I've not written for a month, I've been doing very well. I've been trying to prevent overstraining, including typing discomfort, which is why we did not host Thanksgiving this year. That was a good decision. We had a wonderful time at my sister's home in Miami a few weeks ago.

In honor of such a great weekend with my family, and in the spirit of giving thanks during the holidays, it seems appropriate to document my recent progress. Thanks to the frequent massages, to endocrine balancing efforts, and to my cautious mobility, all of my tight muscles are starting to release their grip. Less muscular tightness has allowed new strengthening efforts, and that has increased my strength. I can again do my usual arm exercises with three pounds of weight, while needing to apply less pressure to the depression just off my shoulder. Keeping my left shoulder down and back (as I walk, sit, cut, or pull) has become second nature after consciously doing it so many times. Although I need to loosen that tension intermittently, otherwise those muscles retighten. The emphasis on my posture has been good; I am moving and sitting with less discomfort.

Older issues are also improving. My lymphedema symptoms have not recurred and there hasn't been another infection scare. The right implant has completely settled in a higher position and will not be requiring surgery. What little scar tissue remained after the ART sessions has dramatically diminished, and frequent massages and stretches are keeping that under control. Even my surgical scars have lightened and are far less noticeable. I have no irregularities of any kind throughout my mastectomy areas, a very reassuring detail.

Day-to-day difficulties are also becoming past history. Sleeping, typing, and driving continue to become more and more comfortable. Even my nerve sensitivity continues to diminish. I can once again shower with warm, although still not hot, water. Toweling after a shower is much less uncomfortable, as is sitting for extended periods of time. I finally have complete range of motion in every direction with both arms, and my left axilla has at last begun to perspire. I can wear most sleeves with *limited* discomfort, even fitted tops! That activity feels luxurious and miraculous. It will never be taken for granted again. One other thing seems different; objects seem to weigh less and less all the time, quite literally. Things that were impossible to lift just a month ago are now possible, although I still need to favor my right arm. Objects actually *feel* lighter.

It seems as though I am once again moving in a direction that makes sense, or at least one with the potential to improve my comfort level. This winter will definitely be better than the last.

2011

CREATIVE REHABILITATIVE EFFORTS

January 4th-6th

I am thrilled to start another year! No, I am not making New Year's resolutions. I am just saying that as far as my rehabilitation, this year might be better. My certainty is based on a wonderful development: the muscles on the left side of my neck have finally disengaged from most motions. Having those muscles more relaxed and being in so little pain are milestones.

In many respects, I might be where I should have been shortly after my initial surgery. Last week I played Ping-Pong with Neil using my left arm. I was amazed. I felt very little pain during and after the game. I also ventured out for a bike ride, an unthinkable activity for nearly two years, and the discomfort was actually manageable. The sense of freedom and joy was overwhelming. I stopped at the park for a joyful cry.

On the other hand, I did not have a plan for what I would do at this point. It had been a dream come true, based on the knowledge that muscular strength can improve years after breast cancer treatment. The concept finally applies. Most of my nerve pain is gone, and the majority of my muscular dysfunction has at last been unraveled. Knowing that my difficulties are stemming from muscular weakness is encouraging. Weak muscles can be retrained and have memory, although I was starting to wonder if mine had Alzheimer's, but they don't. My muscles are finally getting stronger, my arms do not tire as easily, and my limited mobility repertoire is expanding.

Aside from tackling the residual weakness, I need to keep my trapezius muscle from retightening—a somewhat challenging balancing act. I need to be careful and proceed slowly; otherwise the abnormal pattern will return. I will start by avoiding exercises that place my left arm parallel to the ground. At a high angle, my over eager trapezius wants to pitch in more than it should. I started doing leg squats with a five-pound weight loosely held in my hands to ensure my shoulders are not shrugged up. If my shoulders are properly pressed down and rolled back, the activity seems to pull down on the entire neck and shoulder area. The only abdominal exercises I can comfortably perform are upright on an exercise ball, although to understand which muscles *should* be involved, and to keep my shoulder and neck muscles from engaging inappropriately, my hands need to press down on the opposite shoulder.

The various exercises have made my pectoral and back muscles sore. I am not going to let this concern me. Those muscles are frail. They are simply letting me know that I need to add exercises slowly and perform them in a controlled manner.

Professional massages every other week, frequent stretches, endocrine balancing efforts, weekly acupuncture sessions, and daily self-massages loosen most of my muscular tension. I still need rest periods, ice, and I need to be mindful of most movements—it's just rewarding to be making such clear progress. Overcoming most (or at least part) of my pain and weakness might be possible after all.

⸎

MARITAL STRAIN

January 15th-18th

This journal will be incomplete, if I do not make an entry about how my marriage has been uprooted by my cancer diagnosis, and from the lengthy rehabilitation that followed. Our marital difficulties have at least the potential to continue. My rehabilitation is moving in the right direction, but it will take a while.

Perhaps the most important issue, even though I was not aware it was a problem, is how much Sandy resented performing tasks that used to never concern him. He probably thought I would never resume my typical chores. He must have been worried I would no longer be the same partner. I should have guessed some of these concerns; he has been looking very tired and stressed. He could not keep up the enthusiastic momentum he thought he could maintain.

I have been trying to let go of my understandable disappointment. He is only human. No one is perfect, not even him. It has been hard for Sandy to do so much and for so long, and I do appreciate his constancy. Besides, I know he is disappointed at himself for feeling so burdened. I finally understood. If the roles had been reversed, and the difficulties had lasted this long, I would have felt the same way. Although for a while it was hard to be empathetic. His resentment made me feel helpless; I wanted to help him, but I couldn't.

On the upside, we have always been honest with each other, even on issues such as this one, which most people would not be willing to discuss. At the time of that difficult conversation it felt as though we had crossed a bridge that should not have been crossed. The venture paid off. The delayed honesty cleared the air, gave us a better understanding of each other's experiences, and prompted a search for common ground. We learned that there have been many layers beyond the physical challenges that we have both been facing. For a while our focus was on trying to keep our children balanced and ourselves from drowning, in that order of importance. We are continuing to express our feelings without being defensive, always a step in the right direction.

Although, there was still another issue, this one was on the medical management front. Aside from my active medical involvement, Sandy was initially uncomfortable with my complementary approaches. I had been trying to respect his disapproval for the sake of our marital harmony. I tried to understand why he needed to stay so removed from the technical aspects of my care, but I inevitably resented both.

We started moving in the right direction when he read a book that had been on his night table for months: *Breast Cancer Husband: How to Help Your Wife (and Yourself) through Diagnosis, Treatment, and Beyond*. Mr. Silver suggests that breast cancer partners should function as supporters, even if they do not agree with medical decisions. Since needs vary, couples should determine how the well spouse can be of assistance [148]. Sandy realized that his role in my experience has *not* been medical. When he unexpectedly apologized, our medical approaches were no longer an issue.

Sandy's medical disengagement had upsides. It gave me wings to venture towards integrative medical trails; if he had been looking over my medical shoulder, I would not have explored unfamiliar territory. Our different approaches also taught me the importance of respecting traditional medical sensitivities. To avoid discord, I had to consider his perspective.

A glimpse of normality has made him hopeful. Sandy is grateful for the obvious progress, even though he does not understand how it happened. Just last week he said, "I am finally getting my wife back." He at least recognizes that the turning point, in every area, happened when I added complementary approaches.

I am trying to remember that Sandy cannot be part of every new emotion or understand every physical challenge that still lies before me. It's just too hard for him to be so involved. Instead, I've been relying on my support system, my extended family, and on Tatiana in particular. Recently we took the time to acknowledge how beneficial our two-person support group has been. Without it, we would have felt lost.

Our family dynamics have also been transformed. I used to spend most of my time fulfilling Sandy's needs, as well as our children's, but I do not want to revert to those roles. I did it all out of love, and of course I still love my family, I just need to know they can manage without me. I am particularly worried about how Sandy would cope. He is very dependent on me emotionally and domestically, perhaps more than he should be, although he also refuses to contemplate any other way of doing things. That concerns me. I have been reminded that I cannot control my longevity, or even my sense of well-being.

The wish to make my family more independent is not uniquely mine; a first cousin is experiencing a similar sentiment. She confided that feeling so responsible for her grown children is suddenly too much of a burden after her recent breast cancer diagnosis. After acknowledging our need to find a personal agenda, we concluded that encouraging our loved ones to be self-sufficient is just another side of the love coin—it is not abandonment.

⬿⬿⬿

COULD I EVER BE THE SAME AGAIN?

February 6th

I might regain a semblance of the life I once considered normal, although I wonder if I could ever be, or would ever want to be, the same again. I fear going back to unimportant priorities, shed out of necessity during my lengthy rehabilitation.

Scratched from that list is the need to redecorate, unrealistic housekeeping standards, an emphasis on clothes, the need to over exercise, concerns about weight, and the need to control not just my emotions, but those of other people in my life. Rather than seeing what needs to be changed in our house, I try to appreciate the items that symbolize the life we've built together. When the chaos that ensues seems overwhelming, I see it as the price of having a family. If my unfinished chores seem bothersome, I recall the days I could not perform them at all. I don't focus on how stylish my shirts are. I luxuriate in wearing them painlessly. Since I cannot exercise as I once did, I keep in mind that healing from a health crisis can take a long time. Instead of worrying about gaining weight, I try to remember that the ability to do so is a sign of health. If my negative emotions start to brim I no longer turn them away. As soon as I feel the need to control my loved ones, I remember that being in their lives and having them in mine is a privilege. The environment for so much change was created when it took so long to feel well again, therefore on most days, I am grateful for that as well.

During the years I worked as an intensive care nurse I was present when many patients took their last breath. I witnessed how some of them made peace with their loved ones, and with themselves. The forced reprioritizing might have allowed a glimpse at that peace-making experience except unlike them, I have the opportunity to continue living with the insights.

As I go back to my long-neglected distractions, I run the risk of returning to some of my old ways, but that would be a mistake. In many respects, learning those lessons was more important than getting rid of the cancer and rehabilitating. I no longer need to rely on frequent meditations for pain relief, but can I stay in touch with my intuition without them? Can I keep my priorities intact when the gratitude for my timely diagnosis and the sense of appreciation for overcoming so many hurdles fades into the background? I no longer fear dying. I fear living with a sense of regret, with the feeling that I should have done more, or with the impression that I should have done it differently.

～◈～

Setback Urges Chiropractic Care

February 15th-16th

I got too confident. I went a month without a massage and a few days without stretches. The muscles around my neck, which my massage therapist calls *scalenes*, retightened. She reminded me that some of my neck muscles shortened, which is why I've had the discomfort for nearly a year. This now feels like the final frontier that needs to be conquered. My setback and overstraining can be blamed on my wish to do everything I've not been able to do; although clearly, that was a mistake.

I've decided to finally work with a chiropractor. Since massages and stretches loosen most of the muscular tension that caused the cervical compression, it might be possible to address that lingering issue. Besides, he seems familiar with *gradual* muscular rehabilitation.

Strengthening the upper-outer portion of my arms is still the priority, except he modeled a new way to progress without regressing. He stepped on a long band and pulled outwardly, while he slowly rotated his wrist away from his torso. I was given an explanation for something I had already realized through trial and error: to isolate my upper arm muscles, and avoid pain to the depression between my left shoulder and neck, I need to limit the described motion to approximately 30 degrees away from my torso. If done too close to shoulder level, my combined tightness and weakness can create an "impingement syndrome" in the depression just off my left shoulder, although I suppose I already knew that.

My chiropractor reiterated what others have said in the past; I will progress only to a point and then plateau, but that juncture seems difficult to determine. I need to progress and fail, time and time again. I am not there yet; even though the pace is slow my strength is increasing, my pain is still diminishing, and there might be other things I can try and learn. Evidently my present stretches—and perhaps some new ones—will need to become part of the daily repertoire my 50-year-old body now demands, a small price to pay for the comfort they so clearly generate.

If I cannot progress anymore this story will only have a "good-enough ending." But even if no further progress takes place, I've already succeeded. I know to keep my discomfort well under control. I might be more comfortable than others with similar deficits. Those realizations keep me in a constant state of amazement.

⚛

A FATIGUE THEORY

February 25th-30th

It is necessary to elaborate on the adrenal-fatigue topic. The overall sense of well-being, the added strength, and the increased energy are undeniable. Out of necessity I was reminded that aside from their important role with immunity, the adrenal glands help to manage stress. They do that by producing several hormones including epinephrine, norepinephrine, and cortisol [111]. *Cortisol* in particular can become chronically elevated during stressful periods, which can cause weight gain, tiredness, and irritability. With prolonged, extreme, or with repeated stress, low cortisol levels can cause familiar symptoms: weight loss, fatigue, hypoglycemia, and low blood pressure [161,173].

My adrenal glands tried to rally time and time again but they never had a good chance. Before cancer I had sciatic pain for a year, we lost a dear relative to cancer six months prior, Sandy's health had been a concern just the month before, my mother had a cardiac crisis within a couple of weeks, and a dear friend committed suicide the previous month. Given the circumstances my adrenal glands were probably taxed before cancer, although it is more than an assumption. Saliva testing verified low cortisol six months prior. When my integrative doctor identified the problem he suggested an adrenal supplement, except I was not big on nutritional agents. I decided to let nature rebuild my adrenal health—a bad decision. After a cancer diagnosis (and three surgeries) I experienced two years of pain, cancer scares, sleep difficulties, and stressful rehabilitation hurdles.

I've relied on daily inhalers and an annual course of steroids to treat asthma for nearly a decade and a half, but I was unaware that long-term use can cause adrenal insufficiency. Of interest is the asthma attack just two weeks after the double mastectomy. It required a long course of steroids, and after they were discontinued my muscular pain increased.

Perhaps not so coincidentally at around that same time I lost six pounds. The pounds continued to shed. I went from a size six before the diagnosis to a size zero a year later. That size was also getting too large, even though I was eating well and barely exercising. Weakness and weight loss can be symptoms of cancer, including liver cancer, luckily my liver enzymes were normal and my liver was not enlarged. I might be the only woman who has ever been excited, to find a new layer of fat on her lower torso.

Things eased up a bit when my thyroid gland received more replacement, my adrenal glands were probably overworking from that stressor as well.

But since the thyroid and the adrenal glands have a synergistic relationship, the one and a half months of thyroid overstimulation (from the mislabeling) could have triggered the crisis. All of my symptoms correlated with those of very low cortisol levels. I got dizzy when I got up from a lying down position, and even a walk around the block left me exhausted. I could not make it to lunch without a nap, I had to take another one before dinner, and the idea of being away from my bed for the day was incomprehensible. Simple carbohydrates (such as bread and pasta) gave me a headache, made it difficult to think clearly, and made me dizzy for hours. I had to avoid sugar and caffeine, both aggravated the symptoms. Even my rehabilitation was affected by the overmedication setback. I was again exhausted after exercising and my muscles retightened.

I sought endocrine answers. Although, since my thyroid function was back to normal, and because I was having energy and low blood pressure issues, my endocrinologist suggested a cardiologist. To avoid a possibly unnecessary health detour I made an appointment with another endocrinologist, except I had to wait three months for that consultation. By the time I walked into that appointment, the various integrative interventions had been in place for the same length of time. I was pleased. I felt stronger than I had felt in a long time. My (morning) blood cortisol and glucose levels were still low, but they were almost normal.

It seemed necessary to explore what happened to my endocrine system, but the often-impenetrable wall, that divides traditional and integrative medicine, did not allow a clear dialogue. My progress and the adrenal supplement information caused my theory, my symptoms, and my mental health to be questioned by the second endocrinologist. I considered returning with a better explanation and with supporting lab work. But then I realized neither would've served a purpose. He was closed to what had worked; he would never believe there was anything wrong with me. Besides, expecting him to accept my integrative approach, including supplements and acupuncture, would be unrealistic.

In addition, based on what I've experienced, integrative medicine is how I want to approach my endocrine health. My blood pressure has normalized, my energy is improving, and with a reasonable diet the hypoglycemic symptoms are manageable. With the intent of allowing my body to regain its own balance, I've been gradually diminishing the adrenal supplements. That was possible because the lightheadedness is not as noticeable, the headaches have lessened, and I am not as tired. *All* of my muscles are regaining their definition, are less uncomfortable, and are getting stronger. My endocrine issues, including the adrenal imbalance, were having a negative effect on my rehabilitation.

Why do I believe the integrative plan has been working? I have some theories. The combination of exercising less, resting more, a diet with adrenal health in mind, and three months of acupuncture gave my adrenal glands the necessary tools to start recuperating. The active-adrenal supplements, and the thyroid replacement, are also helping by replacing deficiencies.

Progress is undeniable with another acupuncture-targeted problem; my hot flashes are far less frequent. To encourage the improvement I've been avoiding the biggest culprits: caffeine, fried foods, processed flours, sugar, alcohol, chocolate, and fruit before bedtime. Interestingly, all of those are contraindicated for adrenal recovery. Having fewer hot flashes has by extension improved my sleep, which is also important for adrenal health.

Just when I did not think cancer had any more gifts for me, it still had one more. I became aware of an imbalance, which in retrospect was present for a while. This problem, along with the thyroid insufficiency, probably worsened from treatment stressors and very likely interfered with my rehabilitation. Both could have become much bigger problems, even though lifestyle changes and appropriate replacements are very effective.

⚬

OTHERS CANNOT NOTICE PROGRESS

March 11th

No one understands my miraculous milestones, although in all fairness, they did not experience the deficits I did. The lack of outer recognition does not diminish the sense of progress or the pride in the achievement.

Yes, I still look the same, even though the changes are so drastic. People around me are no more able to notice that these days I am in less pain, any more than they could tell when I was in various degrees of it, but again, that is not their fault. Even I cannot see the pain behind my forced smile and my tired eyes, when I look for it in pictures from the last two years.

And yet, the keen observers can notice some things—assuming they carefully scrutinize the situation. Some people could witness how I no longer leave the grocery cart at the end of each aisle, and that I no longer pick up the heaviest items last. A few might notice that I am once again driving my car on a regular basis; for many months my steering wheel was too difficult to maneuver. Others could notice how I can carry more bags at one time, open a few doors with just my left arm, and that on occasion Magic's leash is in my left hand. Even those who receive payments from me might appreciate an important change: my handwriting has improved.

Some changes only I have the luxury of noticing. For a while now, I have been able to press all the soap dispensers in our house with just my left hand. Every time I do it, I am amazed that such a simple motion went from impossible nearly two years ago, to possible but difficult many months later, to completely comfortable now. Only I can tell that I am again becoming left-handed and that I can sleep in any position I want, including my favorite left side, for short periods of time. There is no timetable. I am in no hurry. I will give my body all the time it needs to heal by progressing carefully and gradually, even though no one else will notice.

⌘

REHABILITATIVE GOALS

March 18th

Rather than documenting frustration and setbacks, it is good to finally focus on how my sense of well-being continues to progress. I am feeling less overwhelmed from pain, rehabilitation, and from cancer-related issues. For a while now, I've been trying to accept the likelihood of permanent restrictions, while trying not to close the door on progress. To avoid being upset with the slow pace of my rehabilitation, I removed the pressure of deadlines and the stress of anticipation. I can now confirm that this is a good attitude during unpredictable circumstances.

I am thrilled to document that the muscles around my neck continue to release their grip. The milder discomfort, which still ensues, can usually be massaged and stretched away. As a result, I've finally added the band exercises that were recommended in physical therapy a year and a half ago. Bands allow me to control the resistance based on the type of band I select, and from the distance from which I choose to pull. I either wrap the band around a pole or trap it in a closed door at elbow level. I gradually pull towards and away from my torso in a slow, controlled manner. First I started with a white band, which the first physical therapist explained is the easiest, then within a couple weeks I tried a yellow one, the next level. When I conquered weightless stretches at shoulder level with minimal pain, I started band exercises above and below my shoulders, or as close as my neck muscles allowed. The new angle seems to be strengthening my arm muscles, my pectoral muscles, and many of the muscles that support my shoulders and scapulae. I will increase the band exercises gradually. I do not want another setback. Besides, slow gradual strengthening can lessen the likelihood of lymphedema [140].

My goals remain unchanged. To help relax, reposition, and lengthen short-ened muscles, I will carry on with personal and professional massages. I will continue frequent side-to-side comparisons. I will perform all exercises slowly, with controlled breathing, and with my shoulders pressed down and rolled back. I will stretch daily. To gain more strength I hope to eventually use machines that require simultaneous arm effort. Above all, I will continue to explore new options and believe in my healing potential.

⤜⟡⟐

A MESSAGE FOR OUR CHILDREN

March 20th

Since my rehabilitation will very likely improve in the future, my tale can now be wrapped up with a happier ending than I had envisioned. The idea of no longer journaling brings me back to why I started writing. I needed more than an outlet. I wanted our children to learn from my experience, I just did not want to burden them with every detail in real time.

Therefore this journal entry is for you, Neil and Nicole, and even for you, Andrew. You know that even though you are my stepson, I have loved you like a son from the first day I saw you. Remember, positive or creative ideas might not present themselves if you have a defeated mindset. There is a delicate balance between trying your best and letting go of the need to control situations. Only you will know when to make those judgment calls, don't let anyone make them for you. Your loved ones will not always agree with your approaches, though if they truly love you, they will let you do what is right for *you*.

Physical healing will not always take place, and when it does it might not be as you had imagined, but you can always strive for emotional and spiritual growth. There will always be obstacles and pain, but they are not your worst enemies. If you let them they will teach you a great deal. Never be ashamed of your emotional or your physical scars. Wear them as badges of pride for your well-fought battles. And remember, a well of strength resides within you, but unless you drink from its waters on a regular basis it will remain untapped.

⤜⟡⟐

TIME TO STOP JOURNALING & FOCUS ON LIFE

March 23rd

Today seems like a good day to close the journal. It is the second anniversary of my double mastectomy, and I am closer to achieving what I was hoping to accomplish last year on this very date. I am celebrating my survivorship day cancer-free and with less pain.

Not long ago a breast cancer survivor shared an important sentiment. She believes that many of the breast cancer survivors, who are frequently seen on television and in magazines, are concealing a lot behind their smiling expressions. Those seemingly carefree images create unrealistic expectations in our loved ones, and trying to live up to those standards is overwhelming. She is right. I am not going to say that I will always be happy and grateful to be a breast cancer survivor. That will not always be the case.

It is reassuring to know that I would have still made the same treatment choices, even if I had known what was coming. My goals were to balance my treatment between removing the cancer, lowering the stress associated with annual breast cancer screenings, and avoiding the potential long-term effects of therapies other than surgical. Yes, I am at peace with my chosen treatment, but I would have approached my complications in a different manner.

The proper way to close the journal eluded me for a time. After a while, and thanks to a serial dream, I understood the best approach. To escape recurrent persecution dreams, my mind resorts to another persistent theme: flying. I could never fly for fun, it never worked. Then a few weeks ago I finally did it! I was thrilled! Not just because I was flying without the feeling of persecution, I was doing it with two of my favorite birds leading the way—two red cardinals. The birds flew towards me, they picked me up by the shoulders, and we were immediately air bound. At the time the dream felt very symbolic and quite freeing, even though I did not know what it symbolized. Now I know.

When the last endocrinologist concluded that my symptoms were simply from stress I was disappointed. I felt certain the situation was far more complicated, although he was right on that account. I had not stopped to contemplate the *enormous* role that stress has played in my sense of well-being, as doing so would have felt like a weakness on my part. And yet, feeling so out of control has been more than a growth experience—it has been a significant source of stress. If I really allow myself to go there, the unexpectedness of my cancer was scary; I had been taking care of my health. I've also felt an oppressive sense of responsibility for figuring out my mobility riddle. Then there is the fact that my endocrine system was in such disarray and that it took so long to figure it all out. I am definitely afraid to let my guard down.

And yet, as I think about all that occurred, letting go is exactly what I need to do. I need to trust life, the medical system, and even my own body. My dream was telling me to fully embrace life without allowing fear to intermingle in everything. If I remain in fear it will take away my joy. I need to accept that this phase is finally over, feel free, have fun, and fly, just like I did in my dream. It is time.

Part Four

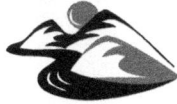

<u>Advocacy</u>

The act of pleading for, support, or recommending; active spousal.

(Dictionary.com)

OUT-OF-THE-BOX AFTERTHOUGHTS

"We must become the change we wish to create."
— Gandhi

"It is not enough to be compassionate. You must act."
— Tenzin Gyatzo

*T*here are two sides to every story, and different approaches to everything, and medicine is no different in that regard. Remember, just like in politics, a healthy debate maintains a balance in medicine, although it is also important to determine how each of us feels about controversial health topics. A good understanding allows us to seek health care providers with similar philosophies.

I have been reminded that every perspective has validity, and not only from the patient's and the practitioners' perspective, but also between different health care providers. Some doctors believe in encouraging their patients to take an active role in their care, while others prefer to make most of the decisions. Some practitioners believe in aggressively pursuing testing after a cancer diagnosis, but others feel it will declare itself. Testing for endocrine abnormalities is not routine, and yet some health care providers feel it is an important aspect of treating middle-age women, or if patients are undergoing cancer therapies. Prescribing physical therapy after breast cancer is not the norm in most offices, although it is in some. Integrative medicine is not endorsed by most health care providers, but those who welcome it would not practice medicine any other way. Most, but not all doctors, believe that annual breast cancer screenings for women under the age of 50 should continue. Many oncologists do not believe that a double mastectomy should be entertained by those of us with an early stage diagnosis if we lack a genetic risk, though others feel it is the patient's call. Some doctors believe in monitoring dense tissue, while their counterparts fear unnecessary screenings and biopsies. Neither skin-sparing nor nipple-sparing mastectomies are endorsed by most breast surgeons, but those who believe in the techniques are passionate about them.

Self-involvement and research can give us a better sense of the different perspectives, which is why I use and explain medical lingo. I truly believe informed patient participation is underexplored. I've tried to include resources written for nonmedical patients, but since it was impossible to exclude medical references, I tried to rephrase the content. In some instances, and for the benefit of those of you who choose to research, I show how my decisions evolved.

It goes without saying that a wealth of breast cancer information is available from the American Cancer Society, the National Institutes of Health, and from the Mayo Clinic, just to name a few sources. I did not focus on their mainstream information. There is a wealth of that already. What I have included is atypical, though possibly useful information and suggestions.

⚜

SELF-ADVOCACY

In addition to rehabilitating, documenting, and researching, I took on another important job after breast cancer; somebody had to piece my complex medical picture together and I was the obvious person to take on that responsibility.

Involvement on this level had not been my style, though I can probably blame this change on cancer as well. It not only gave me more appreciation for life, it left me with a lot of setbacks that were threatening to interfere with my newfound enjoyment. The conflict of interests can prompt some of us to intervene. We want to maximize our health, our sense of well-being, and our comfort level. To make the most of my time with health care providers, I tried to research before appointments. I brought lists so that I would not forget something important, and when I understood their appropriate need, I provided copies of lab work and X-rays from other offices.

Thanks to the internet all of us can access information, including medical journals, which not long ago would have been difficult to obtain. Information is readily available on multiple topics and with different perspectives, but it is important to note dates to ensure currency. Try to sort fact from opinion. Be leery of any source interested in profiting from their claims, particularly if it is not from a reputable health care provider, or if it lacks reliable medical references.

To corroborate findings, I suggest you try to find multiple reliable sources on every topic (i.e., journal articles), and from different perspectives. Websites intended for breast cancer patients, such as www.lbbc.org (Living Beyond Breast Cancer) are a good place to start. You can also access government websites, such as the National Library of Medicine's PubMed/Medline @ http://www.ncbi.nlm. nih.gov/pubmed/. There you can search for a summary (or abstract) of a specific article, which leads to additional citations within the PubMed library. Take advantage of referenced material in text books. If you find it difficult (or expensive) to access full-length medical articles on the internet, you can find most of them in a medical library for a nominal fee.

Blogs are good for sharing emotions, although for treatment advice they can be unreliable, and yet, some experts are effectively reaching out through this medium. Dr. Susan Love's blog at http://blog.dslrf.org/ is a good example. She posts research from important breast cancer meetings and is open to comments. Her foundation supports research to understand *why* breast cancer occurs, rather than focusing on screening methods.

Patient involvement has opened the door for a partnership between patients and doctors labeled *participatory medicine*. The potential benefits of such cooperation are outlined in the 2010 November edition of *American Medical News*, "Has Participatory Medicine's Time Arrived?" The authors highlight that patient-doctor partnerships might be particularly important for chronic diseases, now that medicine has become specialized, and that patients who help to make their health care decisions are more likely to follow recommendations. However, in order to have more input patients need to be well informed and have greater access to their medical records [115]. Through experience, I've learned that this type of cooperation can work particularly well for breast cancer treatments, for rehabilitative issues, and for endocrine issues. In each of those scenarios there are many *right* ways to approach the same problem. Although to maximize our outcomes and our participation, we need to be familiar with *all* of our options, the possible benefits, and *all* of the potential side effects.

Participatory medicine is not for everyone. Not every patient wants to actively research, and not every doctor is interested in having their patients take such an active role. What is important is to find a good match between the two. A patient interested in participating will be disappointed if their doctor is not open to such an option, though the opposite is probably true of a doctor who is hoping for more involvement from their patient.

Limited medical involvement still leaves the need for assistance unaddressed. New careers, such as patient advocates, patient navigators, and concierge medicine, are trying to fill that medical gap. Those practitioners oversee and help coordinate health care decisions, do additional research, help to maximize health care benefits, and assist in the often-difficult search for specialists. Be careful. The industry is so new that there are no uniform licensure requirements, the courses for such certification range significantly, and it still lacks regulation. Some patient advocates have medical backgrounds, while others are more familiar with the insurance industry, among other things. Finding someone with a strong medical background and good personal references might be important for a complex medical issue. However, such personalized assistance, particularly from a doctor, is typically accompanied by a hefty cash-only fee. And yet, the industry is growing very rapidly.

Reputable online advocacy resources are constantly increasing. A large directory of health care advocates, including their background and regional contact information, is the National Association of Health Care Advocacy at nahac.com. For legal, job, or insurance-related issues, a free resource is patientadvocate.org. A few hospitals, although not many, have in-house patient advocates. Some patients are taking participation to new levels. They are creating awareness groups and gathering information for others in a similar situation. One positive example is facingourrisk.org. The website was created for and by women with a genetic predisposition for breast cancer.

On some topics information was not sufficient. I found information gaps on nerve damage, how to rehabilitate from it, as well as limited explanations for lingering fatigue. What I did find would have been difficult to understand without a medical background. Well-meaning, motivated patients are publishing self-advocacy books. Some are extremely helpful, but others seem intent on attacking medical professionals, which in my view creates more health care gaps.

Gladly, medical experts are also writing books and posting information on the internet for those of us who are interested in being informed by reliable sources. Dr. Michael F. Roizen, M.D., Dr. Mehmet C. Oz, M.D., along with The Joint Commission, published, *You the Smart Patient, An Insider's Handbook for Getting the Best Treatment,* a good book on self-advocacy. They remind us that doctors cannot heal us on the spot, and that we should ask informed questions. Information on various types of insurance plans, the complementary-practitioner licensure issue, and self-advocacy resources, are part of the package [136].

Taking the time to understand different medical styles, becoming familiar with our medical dilemmas, and forming cooperative relationships with our doctors can help bridge health care gaps. Dr. Bernie Siegel, M.D., a surgeon by training and a proponent of self-advocacy, states that "exceptional patients do indeed want to be educated and want to be made "doctors" of their own cases." He further adds that "one of the most important roles that they demand of their physicians is that of a teacher." [146]

I was lucky to find that wonderful level of cooperation with most of my health care providers. That openness made them good listeners, encouraged me to keep trying, allowed them to learn from my experience, and made them more willing to readily share their knowledge with me. It created a learning environment from which all of us, including their future patients, can benefit.

⁂

COMPLEMENTARY APPROACHES

Integrative medical practitioners try to combine the best of traditional and complementary medicine to help their patients heal. And even though such an approach will not be recognized in most Western medical settings any time soon, traditional doctors should at least become familiar with integrative approaches within their field. If we try a different approach, it either means traditional medicine let us down in some way, or we cannot afford life-saving treatments. The ability to speak openly and kindly about integrative approaches encourages honesty from patients, which is very important; some patients—particularly cancer patients—inadvertently make inappropriate choices, as they search for a sense of well-being.

My initial plan of action did not include the use of complementary therapies. I only entertained them when traditional medical options felt limited. I did not go at it blindly. I looked for reputable practices and well-trained practitioners with impressive résumés. I researched every supplement and I discussed my approaches with applicable medical providers. I was familiar with integrative medicine, though prior to cancer I was not open to the role that spirituality can play in healing, to energy medicine, or to the use of most supplements, particularly active-endocrine supplements. That is why when things got more complicated, I consulted two endocrinologists.

The holistic approach was enticing. I enjoyed the participatory role that was expected. My integrative physician encouraged me to research and respected my need to adhere to mostly traditional approaches. He explained all of my lab work and gave me copies, while strongly suggesting I too keep detailed records and understand trends. There I found some relief for my premenopausal symptoms with fewer side effects. Although after this experience, I am more than a respectful, close observer, and more than just a believer; I am an advocate for integrative medicine, particularly for cancer patients.

Complementary approaches are gaining ground and experts are taking notice. Some organizations are attempting the necessary, though often difficult, task of creating guidelines. The Mayo Clinic is one, with publications such as the *Mayo Clinic's Guide to Alternative Medicine Second Edition 2011*. The Society for Integrative Oncology (SIO) at www.integrativeonc.org/ displays evidence-based cancer care information. In that website's "clinical corner" section you can find a list of prominent hospitals that offer integrative programs. Breastcancer.org provides information on complementary and holistic medicine, such as how acupuncture might reduce pain, lower fatigue, and control hot flashes [23].

Although undoubtedly, not even those named, reputable organizations would be considered credible sources by those who so fiercely oppose complementary approaches. I understand the hesitation. Research is lacking. As a health care consumer I too would like to see more research, regulation, and oversight. Perhaps the number of us reaching out to those methods, and the finances involved, will compel additional consideration and research. The overwhelming majority of cancer patients, as many as 80%, eventually seek some type of complementary medicine [60].

There is an inverse financial trend between traditional and complementary medicine. In the United States, "Complementary medicine accounts for 600 million office visits a year compared to 350 million total visits to all primary care providers." [75] Medical reimbursements at traditional medical facilities are at an all-time low and are bound to get lower. Patients are less compliant with their financial responsibilities, and reimbursements from insurance companies (and from government health care plans) continue to decline. In contrast, the complementary medical industry is gaining popularity and by extension financial ground. In the United States more cash is spent on complementary and on alternative medicine, than on out-of-pocket medical premiums at traditional medical establishments, including hospitals [60]. Those statistics made me feel less alone. Since I didn't know where else to turn, it was nice to have so much company.

Dissimilar opinions within my marriage, over possible complementary medicine benefits, and over the role that faith can play in healing, have been frustrating, although our opinions have been enlightening from another perspective. Our viewpoints are symbolic of those between Eastern medicine and Western medicine, and if we have found a way to work side by side and respect each other's ideas, then so can those two models. Sandy believes clinical trials and logical explanations should be accessible before any treatment is attempted. I agree. Starting with that approach is absolutely necessary, except I've learned a hard lesson: that data is not always available, and if it is it does not work in every situation. In some instances, non-traditional approaches are more effective.

I could try to gather material on specific complementary therapies. I could quote resources to prove my point for the nonbelievers, but many more capable than me have done that and will continue to do it. Besides, it would be a repeat of what typically happens within my marriage; the believers would find the information validates our shared views, and the nonbelievers would conclude the evidence shaky, and that would reinforce their perspective.

Instead, I would like to pose some questions for you, yes you, the health care professionals who feel integrative approaches have no place in mainstream medicine. I would like to start by pointing out what is already known. You already know that complete healing is not always within your power. You know that because it does not always happen. When it does happen, you don't always understand why it did, any more than you are able to understand how some diseases develop or how a lot of medicines work. You know this because you have experienced time and time again that what works for some patients may not work for others, no matter how hard you try.

I present you with the same dilemma that I posed for my husband the last time we discussed this elusive topic, which now has a lot more middle ground after all he has personally witnessed with me. What then? What happens to those of us who for reasons beyond our control have the atypical complication from the minimally invasive procedure, do not benefit from that often-effective pharmaceutical, do not make progress with the usually helpful therapy, or have a dangerous disease progression that cannot be documented by your rigorous medical standards? They are scary questions; trust me I know, but important ones nonetheless. That is where complementary modalities can play a role. There, the possibility of some improvement can remain, but going there requires a leap of faith on your part, an even more difficult concept to grasp.

Most of the doctors, nurses, and therapists who came in contact with me did more than their best. They let me believe things *could* improve, instead of giving me the statistics about how they usually don't, even though that must have crossed their minds. They knew I was trying unconventional approaches, they listened, and they readily shared their expertise with me. We brainstormed together, and they still let me hope, even when they could not formulate a response. There isn't a billable insurance code for that but perhaps there should be. Many reputable physicians, who believe in some aspect of the integrative medical movement, have seen the importance of allowing the possibility of healing to remain in unlikely circumstances. They might have come to terms with elusive concepts: allowing hope to coexist with uncertainty, and integrating different modalities, might enhance healing potentials.

Merging complementary treatments, herbal supplementation, and Western medicine is the norm in some facilities. A list of centers offering an integrative oncology approach to manage treatment-related symptoms (in the USA), can be found at http://fontherapeutics.com/resources/integrative-oncology-centers/ One such location is the Block Center for Integrative Cancer Treatment in Evanston Illinois, under the direction of Dr. Keith Block, M.D. In *Life over Cancer: The Block Center Program for Integrative Cancer Treatment,* Dr. Block counsels those of us who are interested in trying to prevent a recurrence from a variety of perspectives, including nutrition and endocrine balances [16]. Dr. Block is one of the medical contributors to the breast cancer chapter in *Food and Nutrients in Disease Management.* The text was designed to educate medical students about the role nutrition and supplementation can play in medicine, which is why it is filled with medical research lingo and data [93].

Dr. Jeremy Geffen, M.D., a medical oncologist by training, explored the importance of integrative medicine by having his own integrative cancer center. He is now committed to raising awareness about the positive effects of integrative approaches for cancer care, as he describes in *The Journey Through Cancer: Healing and Transforming the Whole Person.* Dr. Geffen takes into consideration the emotional, the spiritual, and the social aspects of a patient's situation. He believes that we, the cancer patients, need to nurture our bodies by treating them as a "garden" by adding rest, exercise, massage therapy, nutrition, supplementation, yoga, journaling, visualization, acupuncture, chiropractic care, homeopathy, Reiki, and therapeutic touch [60]. More information about his integrative efforts, including details about *The Seven Levels of Healing®,* a program created by Dr. Geffen for cancer patients, can be found on his website: geffenvisions.com.

A long-time leader of the integrative medical movement, Dr. Andrew Weil, M.D., has written *You Can't Afford to Get Sick: Your Guide to Optimum Health and Care.* He suggests that a more integrative approach to medicine would reduce health care costs, might encourage research to understand diseases instead of focusing on masking symptoms, should reduce drug toxicities, and is likely to encourage patients to become more involved in finding solutions. Although, we need to let go of the idea that healing takes place overnight. That mindset results in unnecessary procedures, medicines, and expense. Our present fee-based system is benefitting neither patients nor physicians, though change is taking place. When the book was printed in 2009, nearly a third of all medical schools were "members of the Consortium of Academic Health Centers for Integrative Medicine (www.imconsortium.org)." [170]

In *Healing from the Heart: A Leading Heart Surgeon Explores the Power of Complementary Medicine,* written during his early years as a cardiac surgeon at Columbia's New York Presbyterian Hospital, Dr. Mehmet Oz, M.D., describes a trip to China. There he was shown a model for how Chinese medicine and Western medicine can work side by side. The clinic triaged patients, then sent them to be treated by one of those two medical models. Neither approach was seen as better, or even mutually exclusive. He was told that Western medicine is better for acute problems, and that Chinese medicine might work better for chronic ones [130]. Health care providers interested in understanding how complementary therapies, such as meditation, massages, visualizations and acupuncture can reduce pain, lower stress, and improve outcomes in a clinical setting, particularly in a surgical setting, might be interested in this book.

That clinic in China sounds like a great luxury, and even though I did not have the same experience in the traditional sense of the word, my endocrine and rehabilitative treatment still combined the two approaches, a merging that worked quite well in my situation.

I propose that just like we your patients need to understand that you are not always able to predict outcomes, and heal us exactly when we want you to heal us, that you too consider contemplating the world of possibilities beyond your preconceived medical restraints, for the sake of your patients' healing potential. Particularly when all else has failed, or if your patient is not yet ready for a riskier approach. The concept might be a possibility even if you are not a believer—your wish to help others heal is why you do what you do. Go ahead, take a chance, you were never meant to understand everything, but it does require a leap of faith on your part and you too would have to go off your preconceived medical mentality trail. That is the only way to explore unfamiliar medical horizons.

THE ENDOCRINE PAIN-FATIGUE CONNECTION

It is not yet known why so many women continue to experience various degrees of pain after breast cancer treatment, while many others do not, having undergone the same therapies [133], but as a rule, endocrine issues are not considered a contributing factor. One risk factor seems to be pain in other parts of the body [59,103]. Prior to cancer I had daily headaches and persistent back pain, and both were dramatically lessened with endocrine balancing efforts. On the other hand, the connection between muscular pain and weakness as a result of specific endocrine imbalances is well documented, even for mild thyroid deficiencies, although not all of those patients experience these difficulties.

Without consistent medical validation I considered excluding the endocrine topic, but careful consideration allowed it to remain. First, the high incidence of breast cancer and hypothyroidism must cause overlaps. Up to 7% to 10% of older women might have subclinical hypothyroidism [92], and as many as a quarter of us develop hypothyroidism during or before menopause [127]. Many of us don't know that we have the condition, and half of us who do have it develop adrenal insufficiencies [138]. Adrenal imbalances can result from severe and repeated stress, and cancer certainly fits that criteria. The information gap among physicians, and the treatment variations between traditional and integrative practitioners, might complicate or delay an endocrine diagnosis. Due to the possible overlaps I feel compelled to share how I found some pain relief, how my fatigue was diminished, and how my mental-clarity issues were lessened, even though my approaches will not be helpful for all survivors with similar symptoms.

The endocrine system is a checks-and-balances system. Specific glands, including the adrenal and the thyroid gland, compensate for one another when that becomes necessary. Over time, and if the initial problem cannot correct itself, other imbalances might follow, especially during prolonged and stressful circumstances. Since our bodies are bound to have a similar response to stress, regardless of the stressor [111], adjusting abnormal thyroid and cortisol levels might provide some relief. Excessive fatigue and mental-clarity difficulties can result from many cancer therapies, from anemia, from poor nutrition, or from dehydration, just to name a few causes, but they are also symptoms of hypothyroidism [143] and of low cortisol levels [111]. Hot flashes are usually the result of low estrogen levels, but hypothyroidism might worsen them; the thyroid gland plays a role in temperature regulation [89].

Stress hormones, including cortisol, could fluctuate through treatment. A cancer diagnosis and the physical strain from treatment might cause abnormally high cortisol levels, which could cause weight gain, fatigue, and mental clarity difficulties. Cortisol levels might drop with the stress of prolonged treatment or when steroids, which sometimes accompany chemotherapy, are discontinued. In this section I will explain why steroid use or the sudden discontinuation can cause low cortisol levels, although clearly, I received steroids for a different reason. Chronically low cortisol levels could explain why some cancer patients overcome their fatigue after a few months, and why others continue to experience it for years.

Surgical menopause, medical menopause, steroid use, and stress, can interfere with normal thyroid function [145]. Radiation in proximity to the thyroid gland, and poor nutrition due to chemotherapy, might affect thyroid function directly or indirectly; patients undergoing cancer treatments should have thyroid screenings twice a year [138].

Remember, from a *traditional* medical perspective, specific supplements and hormones are contraindicated for breast cancer survivors. Since they might stimulate cancer growth directly or indirectly, traditional physicians recommend that all sex hormones, or anything capable of producing them, are avoided, even by women with a history of ER-negative breast cancers (not fueled by estrogen). *All* of us are at a higher risk of a second cancer, and the second one might have different characteristics. The hormones that need to be avoided include, but are not limited to, testosterone, pregnenolone, and DHEA. DHEA might encourage estrogen and testosterone production [60], it is readily available without a doctor's prescription, and it is often present in adrenal supplements. If taking anti-estrogen therapy, all supplements and herbs typically used to treat menopausal symptoms should also be avoided. Even some prescription drugs, such as select antidepressants, might weaken anti-estrogen therapy. Webmd.com is a website intended for nonmedical health consumers. It has a broad listing of prescription medicines, herbs, and supplements, along with a list of possible interactions.

But endocrine balance is about more than just comfort and quality of life. Even though not all studies have arrived at the same conclusion, some experts believe that postmenopausal women with hypothyroidism (and very specific abnormal thyroid markers) might have an elevated breast cancer risk [95,157]. The connection is not well understood, but thyroid hormones seem to influence estrogen metabolisms [157]. High cortisol levels from repeated stress have been associated with a higher incidence of breast cancer, perhaps because cortisol plays an important role in mammary gland development and function [5]. Select doctors believe that altered cortisol levels (including high and chronic low levels), which can cause poor sleep, abnormal body weight, and irregular glucose metabolisms, can create a negative endocrine terrain that might increase the likelihood of a cancer recurrence [16].

Excluding the endocrine aspect would support the *main* thing I feel is wrong with our health care system—compartmentalized information, treatment, and thinking. Without my medical records, both endocrinologists were unable to realize that I had been experiencing hypothyroid and hypoadrenal symptoms for years. Compartmentalized thinking kept the pain specialist from considering the endocrine issue, which might have made a difference with my pain and rehabilitation at an earlier juncture. Such approaches can be problematic; our bodies are not made up of separate compartments. They are like a typically harmonious orchestra that cannot perform well when one player is out of tune.

Pay close attention, some of you might be experiencing similar symptoms. The combination of thyroid and adrenal imbalances increased my muscular pain, interrupted my sleep, made it hard to think clearly, and made exercising either difficult or impossible. Under normal circumstances sleep and exercise do the opposite: they lower stress and increase energy.

My search for endocrine answers began when I was trying to understand my atypically high blood pressure. The unwelcome investigations taught me the importance of getting thyroid imbalances under control for cardiovascular health. Hypothyroidism can disturb blood flow [92], even in individuals with mild hypothyroidism [101], and it can cause both hypotension [145] and hypertension [150,165]. "Hypothyroidism reduces the amount of nitric oxide in the lining of the vessels, causing them to stiffen." [53] L-Arginine, a nitric oxide precursor [47], not only lowered my blood pressure, it made my muscles feel like they had breathed fresh air.

My curiosity was sparked. I began to suspect that some of my muscular pain could be from hypothyroidism. Verification took a while. My first hint was in an article published in *Clinical Endocrinology*, where the researchers concluded that thyroid replacement might improve "neuromuscular dysfunction" [114]. Additional information fueled the theory. I confirmed the deficiency can cause muscular pain and muscular weakness [87]. I understood how hypothyroidism can contribute to numbness and nerve pain [113,128], how it can lower exercise tolerance [29], and that in rare instances, it can cause muscular wasting [87]. I knew I was on the right track.

Adrenal health is also important. Under functioning adrenal glands can cause muscular weaknesses [161], which might explain why my overall muscular pain increased six weeks after I started addressing the thyroid issues. In time I learned that to increase thyroid replacement doses, it might be necessary to address low cortisol levels as well [19]. If thyroid medication is taken when an adrenal insufficiency is present, symptoms can worsen [149]. That is exactly what happened to me, although to an extreme, from the unknown, excessive thyroid replacement.

Most traditional medical practitioners, and most traditional medical literature, do not recognize adrenal insufficiencies until they are more advanced, nor believe in integrative approaches to test or treat the condition [173]. Traditional doctors check cortisol levels with a one-time morning blood level, while integrative physicians prefer to rely on saliva testing at different times over a 24 hour period. That gives a sense of an individual's cortisol pattern, which tends to rise and fall throughout the day.

Since they generally prescribe different pharmaceuticals, they also differ in how they approach hypothyroidism. Traditional endocrinologists usually prescribe a *long-acting* version of the deficient thyroid hormone, a T4 *synthetic* replacement. They believe our bodies are capable of converting that into the *short-acting* T3 hormone. Integrative endocrinologists usually prescribe a combination of long- and short-acting thyroid hormones, from *desiccated animal* glands. They believe the combination is a little more similar to human thyroid hormones. In my opinion both approaches work in different situations. When it felt like my adrenal hormones were very low, and since cortisol is needed for thyroid hormone conversion [149], I felt better on a combination of the long- and the short-acting thyroid hormones. Then, when my symptoms were suggesting that my cortisol levels were higher, I did better with the long-acting type.

The two groups might treat different symptoms and lab ranges. Integrative doctors are more likely to explore additional endocrine treatment in patients with normal TSH levels if tiredness, weight gain, depression, mental fogginess, and muscular pain are not resolved. Some traditional physicians overlook higher TSH levels, which in lab reports is considered normal in the 5.0 range, even though in 2003, the American Association of Clinical Endocrinologists recommended doctors aim for TSH levels of 0.3 to 3.0 [145]. Everyone is different, but I felt better when my TSH reached .7. The two groups could start by referring patients to each other when their approach is not working. Research between them would also be educational, though unlikely.

Some chiropractors have tried to bridge those gaps by offering supplements to their patients. That might work for mild endocrine imbalances, but for more complicated scenarios an integrative M.D., a traditional endocrinologist, or an integrative endocrinologist might be more appropriate. They have broader knowledge, plus the ability to order labs and prescribe.

Hydrocortisone is what traditional endocrinologists prescribe for an advanced adrenal insufficiency. Yes, steroids at low doses are recommended, even though they can cause endocrine suppression at higher doses or in repeated quantities. But Hydrocortisone is very different—it is at least 5 times less powerful than Prednisone [149]. Hydrocortisone has *bio-identical* properties to cortisol (similar in makeup), which is why integrative physicians steer away. They believe the similar properties can create an endocrine dependency; thus weaning from them might be more challenging.

Adrenal glandular extracts, which have been used since at least the 1930s for various conditions, are the recommended treatment for an adrenal insufficiency by integrative doctors. Although, since they are made from animal adrenal glands, they might contain *aromatase* enzymes capable of converting into postmenopausal estrogen. As far as I can tell this is simply a theory. Adrenal glandular supplements need further research—the mechanism of action is not well understood [111]. It is unclear how they might affect those of us with a history of breast cancer. Most medical information, including data between breast cancer and endocrine issues, is also compartmentalized. Many of us with more than one health problem find it difficult to juggle them safely.

Nonetheless, supplements should be handled with care. Many, including adrenal glandular products, have very active ingredients. Adrenal glandular supplements should only be taken when absolutely necessary, and then only in the lowest possible amounts. Their appeal lies in their ability to stimulate the adrenal glands by providing cortisol-like ingredients. On the other hand, glandular extracts from *ovarian or uterine* sources should definitely be avoided. Those are more likely to encourage female hormone production in larger amounts. Try to research every ingredient in every supplement. Glandular products should be used with the supervision of a physician familiar with them (even though such physicians are hard to find); unnecessary use can suppress the adrenal glands or cause unwanted hormones.

All of that explains why from the perspective of my breast cancer history, I was hesitant to try adrenal glandular supplements, but my cortisol levels must have been very low; I was having difficulty functioning for more than one hour at a time and rest was not restorative. The dizziness, heat and light sensitivity, low blood pressure, and the symptoms of low blood sugar were making me feel like I was spiraling into a very bad place. I was trying to stay out of the emergency room. I wish I had known that cortisol saliva kits are available from reputable companies on the internet without a doctor's prescription. I did not. I only had my symptoms to guide me. I did what would have been done in a traditional medical setting: I treated the crisis at hand and as soon as I could, I removed the conflicting element.

It was a good trade-off. The supplements, along with the lifestyle changes I had already been attempting, provided undeniable improvement. I used the adrenal glandular supplements in the lowest possible amounts and weaned myself from them as soon as I could. After just a few months my adrenal glands started bouncing back. Since they eventually allowed aggressive exercise to help prevent a recurrence, their long-term benefit is bound to outweigh possible short-term negative effects. Exercise might lower breast cancer recurrences, particularly in postmenopausal women [94].

If Hydrocortisone is used for extreme adrenal fatigue, the pharmaceutical might be needed for months [19], although the same applies to adrenal supplements. Both should be withdrawn carefully and slowly, a juggling that requires a lot of self-involvement. In addition, "once adrenal fatigue seems under control, it's sometimes necessary to adjust the thyroid hormone supplement." [138] Neither Hydrocortisone nor adrenal supplements are long-term measures, unless the adrenal glands can no longer produce cortisol (Addison's disease). Hydrocortisone is then necessary for life. In light of my breast cancer history, and since Hydrocortisone is less likely to encourage postmenopausal estrogen production, I would have preferred low-dose Hydrocortisone over adrenal glandular extracts to treat my adrenal insufficiency; although for that, I would have needed traditional medical validation.

Gladly, most adrenal insufficiencies do not require such active measures. The majority of people with adrenal insufficiencies have less acute, but more debilitating symptoms that become the norm. Some of those respond well to lifestyle and dietary changes, and to stress-reduction techniques. Meditation, yoga, tai chi, humor, biofeedback, and additional rest can all help. Exercise programs should be increased *gradually*. Over-exercising through an adrenal insufficiency might over tax the endocrine system [149]. The strain could lead to more fatigue, rather than less, as should be the case with exercising.

From an integrative perspective, adding moderate amounts of vitamin C, homeopathic remedies, vitamin E, and B vitamins, particularly B6, might be important with adrenal insufficiencies [173]. Eating frequent meals (starting with breakfast), and adding fresh fruits, vegetables, protein, and complex carbohydrates, can go a long way. Avoiding caffeine, alcohol, refined sugars, and fried foods might make a difference [173]. Specific *adaptogenic* herbs (herbs that adjust to what the adrenal glands need) can also be helpful [111], although I suggest researching those to personalize treatment. One example is licorice root. The root can help stabilize cortisol levels, but it might also raise blood pressure [149]. In my experience, acupuncture can also play an important role in endocrine balancing efforts. Again, it is important to research, find a practitioner familiar with these approaches, and take into consideration all aspects of your medical history. What worked for me might be contraindicated for someone else.

One of the only traditional medical articles I found on adrenal insufficiencies was posted by the U.S. Department of Health and Human Services, in cooperation with the National Institutes of Health, and the National Institute of Diabetes and Digestive and Kidney Diseases, "Adrenal Insufficiencies and Addison's Disease." I had the most common symptoms: chronic, worsening fatigue; muscle weakness; loss of appetite; and weight loss. I also had 80% of the "less-common" ones [161]. An adrenal insufficiency might not be noticed until significant stress, such as surgery [173]. However, it can be temporary if addressed in time.

My adrenal insufficiency could have occurred for reasons other than stress. *Secondary adrenal insufficiency*, a condition that can result from steroid use, could have been part of the problem. Secondary adrenal insufficiency can suppress ACTH production in the *pituitary* gland, and that in turn limits adrenal function, because ACTH is necessary for cortisol production, among other things [161]. Limited adrenal *and* pituitary function can cause a lot of problems. Both glands are important for proper stress responses during infections, cancer treatments, surgeries, and post-operative pain, just to name a few stressors. This insufficiency used to be rare but it is becoming more prevalent. The use of steroids for a variety of reasons, including the higher incidence of asthma, continues to increase.

The suspicion was confirmed when I got another asthma attack. If you experience similar symptoms when your steroids are lowered or discontinued, adrenal suppression might be playing a role in your muscular pain and fatigue. As was the case with the asthma episode after the double mastectomy, my muscular discomfort and fatigue increased when I tried to wean myself from steroids. In retrospect,

I had experienced difficulties weaning myself from steroids for years, and I was exhausted for months afterwards.

I did not share the scenario with the second endocrinologist to discredit his work on my case. I included it because it is symbolic of how lack of communication between patient and doctor, doctor to doctor, and between traditional practitioners and integrative physicians can interfere with medical care. We did not know each other, and we walked into the exam room with very different beliefs; he that only traditional methods can manage and test endocrine issues, while I was sensing otherwise.

Since I was not yet aware they could be transferred, the lack of medical records presented a bird's eye view of the problems. We did have the history and physical page, although that only included *present* medications and symptoms. The month before I stopped the daily inhalers that I had been taking for years, but the gathered information did not reflect the change. My annual course of steroids was also absent. I was not taking steroids at the time, but they can have a negative effect on adrenal health for months afterwards. He was looking for high cortisol levels and weight gain. He would not find those. I had been there years before that day, had gone to the other extreme a few months before, and thanks to the integrative efforts, my adrenal health had improved. My (morning blood) cortisol and blood pressure were still low, but almost normal, and I was still very thin. I could not help—I did not understand my medical puzzle.

I eventually understood. Aside from how difficult it is to share medical records, doctors seldom speak with one another when a referral is made. His conclusions were based on the information available to him and because of his traditional medical perspective. On the other hand, my symptoms had been real. The results from my integrative approaches were undeniable.

Unrecognized endocrine difficulties have prompted a medical movement in books, websites, and blogs. Almost every thyroid resource includes some information about the adrenal glands—they are that interconnected.

Some advocates have been inspired by their own struggles. *Overcoming Adrenal Fatigue* by Kathryn Simpson, MS, is the result of personal experience and research. The book has patient stories, questionnaires, and many practical suggestions [149]. In *The Menopause Thyroid Solution*, Ms. Mary Shomon, also an endocrine patient, describes how symptoms from hypothyroidism, perimenopause, and from menopause are alike and develop during similar life stages, making an adequate diagnosis difficult. Even women who are not overweight might suffer from hypothyroidism [145]. In my opinion, this book is a must for any woman who has been diagnosed with (or suspects) hypothyroidism. Ms. Shomon compiled a list of doctors from different states on her website. Those practitioners come highly recommended by patients who have struggled with endocrine imbalances, particularly with hypothyroidism. At http://thyroid.about.com/cs/doctors/a/topdocs.htm, you can find that unusual information. I can't speak for all of them, but there I found an integrative concierge physician with a good endocrine understanding.

Integrative health care providers are also making important contributions. Dr. Michael Lam, MD., MPH., @ www.DrLam.com, explains adrenal fatigue in detail. *Thyroid Balance, Traditional and Alternative Methods for Treating Thyroid Disorders,* by Dr. Glenn S. Rothfeld, M.D., M.Ac., and Ms. Deborah S. Romaine, explains thyroid diseases, has a chapter on adrenal insufficiencies, and it mentions how cancer treatments can affect those balances [138]. Another book with a traditional and an integrative approach is *Thyroid Power: 10 Steps to Total Health*, by Richard L. Shames, MD., and Karilee H. Shames R.N., Ph.D., although this book is a little different. It highlights that adrenal imbalances happen *gradually*—like Hans Selye's general adaptation syndrome. Adrenal treatment should be based on the stage the patient is experiencing [143].

That brings me to an important point. Since some supplements lower cortisol levels and others raise them, understanding the adrenal insufficiency *stage* is crucial for proper treatment. Trying to understand these issues can be daunting, that is why I am giving a brief overview. It is not an easy task and a lot of trial and error is involved, but living with endocrine imbalances is more difficult. Improvement does not happen overnight and a lot of lifestyle changes are needed, but an improved sense of well-being could be the reward. Even symptoms as severe as fibromyalgia and chronic fatigue might benefit from adrenal nutrition and supplementation [93].

In early 2011 asthma again came knocking on my door for what I thought was its usual early-spring allergic annual visit, when every oak tree in the state of Florida is pollinating. As I tried to wean myself from the steroids, I experienced the familiar muscular pain and the undeniable fatigue. Because my endocrine system cannot balance itself as readily as it should, I slowly tapered the steroids and I lowered my physical activity. Unlike previous years, I resorted to active-adrenal supplements and I relied on acupuncture. The results were encouraging. My stamina was better, my muscles were not as uncomfortable, I needed fewer steroids, and I got over the asthma in a shorter period of time. The milder asthma attack makes sense from an integrative medical perspective: under-functioning adrenal glands can lower immunity, worsen asthma, and increase allergies [149].

But I knew if I continued needing an annual course of steroids and two daily inhalers, my hard-earned progress would be hard to maintain—my endocrine suppression would continue. I went on a respiratory-health quest to lower my asthma symptoms with integrative measures, although again, complex situations do not have magic bullets. The *combination* of different measures is what made a difference. I started by pursuing allergy testing. I was experiencing asthma-like responses to allergic triggers, such as oak pollen, but to my surprise the test was completely negative. The next step was a speech therapy referral. My asthma specialist wanted verification for what he suspected was *vocal cord dysfunction* (VCD). VCD is defined as abnormal vocal cord tightening that can mimic or worsen asthma, and can be confirmed (as mine was) by laryngoscopy. In speech therapy I learned that specific visualizations, relaxation techniques, and appropriate stretches can help manage VCD. Although, asthma inhalers might worsen VCD; if both are diagnosed, nebulizers might be more appropriate.

When the above measure helped but with room for improvement, I took into consideration a magnesium deficiency, as is entertained in integrative literature when muscle cramps and constipation accompany asthma [93]. Intravenous magnesium has been used to treat children during acute asthma attacks, but while some physicians believe in the benefits, not all do. If you are interested in exploring how this deficiency might increase bronchial spasms, cause migraine headaches, interfere with sleep, how fatigue syndromes and nerve disorders can be worsened by it, and how poor diet and stressful situations might exasperate it, you might want to read *The Magnesium Miracle* by Dr. Carolyn Dean, M.D., N.D. [42]. If needed, as was the case in my situation, appropriate magnesium supplements might lower muscular pain and improve exercise tolerance [16].

While I am on the subject of minerals, calcium is also important for neuromuscular health. The excess of either calcium or magnesium can cause a deficiency in the other, and both might be reduced by some medications, including steroids, aging, and by specific endocrine imbalances. We all know calcium is important and easily found in food sources. What most of us don't know is that magnesium (which is needed for calcium absorption), is hard to measure or obtain through diet alone.

The combined efforts, including VCD management, adrenal interventions, acupuncture, along with limited outdoor exposure during peak oak blooming season, might explain why in the spring of 2012—and for the first time in 15 years—I did not have my usual spring asthma attack. I've not needed steroids, antihistamines, short-acting inhalers, or long-acting inhalers, for over two years!

You are probably thinking that this time I really ventured into a completely unrelated trail, but not really. Everything in our bodies is interconnected. To balance risks and benefits it might be necessary to look at the entire picture. Fewer steroids have helped my adrenal health, my sense of well-being and by extension my quality of life. Since my endocrine system is not as suppressed, I need less adrenal support, I've gained weight, and I can exercise regularly. The adrenal diet, which limits alcohol, fried foods, red meat, and refined sugars, is also good for my cardiovascular health, as is my normal blood pressure. Regular exercise, improved sleep, and such a healthy diet are my most important weapons against cancer.

Even now, I cannot contemplate popular breast cancer survivor activities. My exercise tolerance is better, but I still don't have the strength to keep up with breast cancer survivors who row regularly, and I lack the stamina for a three day walk. That is not surprising. Even though they have improved, my mid-day and afternoon saliva cortisol levels are still low. Recovering from a prolonged adrenal insufficiency can take a while. What I have is more energy than I had for four years, clearer thinking, diminished hot flashes, fewer headaches, improved muscular strength, better sleep, and hardly any muscular aches.

My adrenal condition, which had probably been present for years to a lesser extent, does not officially exist. I did not have a traditional lab test to document it, and I was not treated by a well-researched pharmaceutical. That is a good thing. To get that validation I would have needed a serious endocrine crisis, or a dangerous and possibly inconclusive test. From an insurance preexisting condition perspective, the lack of medical documentation is also beneficial.

I will carry on with an integrative approach. To lessen future asthma attacks, I will follow traditional medical suggestions. With the intent of obtaining optimal endocrine balance, with a focus on nutrition and lifestyle changes, I will continue to work with an integrative physician. I will try to limit the use of endocrine supplements, keep my stress in check, and I will remain meticulous with my diet.

As you can see, you too might need to think outside the box to help determine how other aspects of your health are increasing your pain, prolonging your fatigue, and interfering with your sense of well-being. Cancer treatment, and the associated stress, can have a negative effect on preexisting conditions or cause new ones.

Listen to your body, research, and keep looking for answers! But remember, many supplements and homeopathic medicines can interfere with the benefits of chemotherapy. Some are contraindicated for specific health problems, and all of them need to be discontinued several days before surgery. To help understand possible supplement/therapy conflicts, an oncology dietician is often available in cancer centers. East can meet West if self-advocacy, participatory medicine, and if traditional and integrative approaches are combined in an informed manner.

⟿⟿

PAIN AFTER BREAST CANCER TREATMENT

Before we can try to find relief, we need to look for a way to describe our pain. It is important to understand patterns, realize which activities are limited or impossible, get a sense of whether the discomfort is improving or worsening, and explain what has or has not helped. "Studies have shown that the more detailed those descriptions are, the better physicians are at pinpointing the source of pain and administering appropriate treatment." [15] Although remember, no therapy can accelerate or create nerve healing. Only time and our innate ability to heal can accomplish those goals minimally, partially, or completely. For now, the only medical goal is to ease symptoms.

It is difficult to know how many women in the United States are experiencing pain after breast cancer—different studies have arrived at different conclusions. Besides, as was the case in my situation, muscular imbalances and intense nerve pain might worsen over time. Pain is difficult to measure. A standard way has not been established, although in 2005 Dr. M. Leidenius, M.D., Ph.D., published a questionnaire within a medical article that can serve as a guide [100].

Pain is a broad term. Breast cancer survivors are experiencing different types of pain, including phantom pain, which can be either short- or long-term. For long-term pain, including pain from metastases and unresolved nerve pain, prescription medicines are very important. Upper-arm pain and cervical compressions are considered "common" among breast cancer patients, and both can weaken shoulder and upper-arm muscles [153]. Scar tissue, from either surgery or from radiation, can cause pain by limiting movement in skin, muscles, and/or tendons. It can also entrap nerves and cause painful *neuromas* [17]. Aside from massages, surgery is another way to reduce scar tissue. Frozen shoulders, another common side effect, usually improve with proper movement, though if that is ineffective, surgery might be necessary. Any type of pain might make us fear a recurrence, but that is usually not the cause.

Since every treatment can cause pain, the combinations of several interventions increases the likelihood of pain. Chemotherapy can cause distant nerve pain (*peripheral neuropathy*) in areas such as hands and feet. Radiation can worsen or cause chronic pain [133,142], and lymphedema can happen from lymph node removal, particularly if the area receives radiation [81]. If radiation causes pain on the skin (*topical*), you might need to avoid products with aluminum, alcohol, or perfumes. Muscular trauma from radiation might not be felt for months or even years, but typical mobility suggestions can help.

Muscular pain (or joint pain) can also be caused by aromatase inhibitors, or when we get into the habit of sitting or standing with our back hunched and our shoulders leaning forward (*protective posturing*). All of us, who had any type of breast cancer surgery or treatment, might sit or stand in that manner without realizing the consequences.

If muscular imbalances develop as a result of breast cancer surgery, the pectoral muscles are usually affected first. Breast reconstructions can cause muscular pain by stressing the pectoral, shoulder, neck and back muscles, but stretching and strengthening those muscles can lessen it [31].

So much strain can cause trigger points in the trapezius muscle. Trigger points in the trapezius might develop from "overload, compression, and trauma," and since the trapezius is the main muscle that supports the weight of the arms [52], nerve disruptions to an arm can inadvertently stress the trapezius muscle. "Of all the muscles in the body, the trapezius is the one most commonly afflicted with trigger points." [40] Though in general, breast cancer literature does not address how this muscle is affected. Keep in mind that even though the trapezius muscle is large, superficial, and easy to examine, different neck, shoulder, and back muscles can cause pain after breast cancer treatment. You need to figure out which ones need to be relaxed and strengthened, either underneath or in the vicinity of the trapezius.

Areas from where tissue is transferred might also be afflicted with muscular weakness. Survivors who chose a muscular graft reconstruction need to know which muscles were repositioned, how that affects mobility, the best ways to stretch, how massages can help, and how to compensate [81]. All of that can be accomplished by researching and by consulting with experts, but again, paying attention to individual sensations is important. Not everyone has such issues, and the extent of the difficulties, when they do occur, can vary from woman to woman.

Overall, the frequency of chronic *nerve* pain after breast-conservation surgeries and after mastectomies might be similar [78]. Either way, the likelihood increases when a lot of lymph nodes are removed (ALND) [103]. Damage to the *intercostobrachial nerve* is a common culprit [17,169]. Surgeries that "spare" the intercostobrachial nerve can lower the incidence of nerve pain, but other nerves might also be affected [78]. Nerve injury can cause pain and unusual sensations to the chest, axilla, and to the affected arm. An understanding of which nerves provide sensation to the muscles that are experiencing sensory deficits might help determine a course of action. The understanding led me to believe that in my case, a posterior branch of the *axillary nerve* might have been affected. Biofeedback, transcutaneous nerve stimulators, immobilization of the affected arm, acupuncture, and pharmaceuticals might lower nerve pain, but symptoms stemming from nerve damage can be "severe and difficult problems to treat." [107]

A couple of articles set me on the right track. "Post Breast Therapy Pain Syndrome" (PBTPS), at www.cancersupportivecare.com/neuropathicpain.php, describes how different therapies can cause nerve pain and frozen shoulders, how pain syndromes are underreported and misunderstood, and which pharmaceuticals might help [142]. If you are looking for nerve pain validation, explanations, and suggestions on how to discuss this seemingly obscure topic with your health care providers, a good place to start is "Post Breast Therapy Pain Syndrome Handout" at cancerlynx.com/pbtpshandout.html [169].

Pain specialists can determine if there is nerve damage, they can prescribe pharmaceuticals, and they can diagnose a muscular dysfunction. They can also do nerve blocks and trigger point injections. Those common treatments for nerve pain could have allowed better posture and eased some of my nerve pain, but neither would have prevented muscular imbalances. Since some muscles could not perform their intended task, others would have still compensated. Nerve blocks also have their own set of possible complications, and I had already experienced my fair share. Even if a pain specialist identifies the problem, as mine clearly did, he or she does not carry out suggestions. Mine ordered electrical stimulation (also called a TENS unit), which can help manage nerve pain [107], but it was not available at the recommended facility. I did not insist. I was not familiar with the possible benefit.

Since *acute* pain after surgery seems to increase chronic pain [133], nerve blocks at the time of surgery might reduce the incidence for as long as a year [82]. I was starting to contemplate nerve blocks after my second physical therapy attempt. I believed my pain specialist when he told me that the nerve pain cycle needed to be broken before it became self-sustaining.

It does sound like an archaic idea, and it is not for everybody, but I let my nerve and my muscular pain guide me towards what I needed to do and away from what I should not do. I was afraid to lose the ability to differentiate between those innate mechanisms with a nerve block. The approach is not always appropriate. Just like muscular pain, nerve pain can also be referred or felt in a different area. I stayed away from aggressive procedures for reasons other than fear of complications. I knew nerves can be compressed by scar tissue [153,171], and I theorized that extreme muscular tension was contributing. As it turns out, addressing both lowered my nerve pain.

And yet, pain was a great guide. It taught me the difference between a tight muscle and scar tissue. I learned when an area needed to be massaged, if it needed rest, if it benefitted from heat, or when it needed to be iced. Pain also guided my rehabilitation. It was obvious when a muscle had been overworked and when it had been stretched in the proper manner. Having less pain meant I was doing something right. When my irregular nerve sensations began to change and then improved, I understood that nerve healing was trying to take place. If nerve pain was involved and massages worsened pain in a specific area for days, then I needed to avoid direct pressure.

I did not believe I would have this old-fashioned approach validated in literature, but I was proven wrong. I read the chapter "Pain is Not the Ultimate Enemy" in Mr. Norman Cousins' *Anatomy of an Illness*. Mr. Cousins graciously describes the wisdom of pain. To illustrate how complete lack of pain can be problematic, he presents individuals with leprosy. They injure themselves because they cannot feel pain. This uplifting book recounts Mr. Cousins' use of participatory medicine, self-advocacy, adrenal support, and humor to lessen stress and heal the adrenal glands [37].

I'm not suggesting needless suffering. We are all different. The answers are as individual and as complex as the problems that prompted them. Different pharmaceutical combinations might help, although you might need to persevere until the right dose and type are found. With fewer side effects, I would have continued one of the four medicines I tried. My intolerance might have stemmed from hypothyroidism. I've since learned that thyroid levels should be monitored if specific steroids, antidepressants, or select anticonvulsants (typically used for the treatment of nerve pain) are prescribed. Some of those pharmaceuticals might be metabolized differently in individuals with hypothyroidism, causing increased hypothyroid symptoms or medication side effects [145]. In time *Topical* (applied to the skin) Ketamine and Amitriptyline provided short nerve pain reprieves. Pharmaceutical approaches are often inadequate for the treatment of nerve pain [126], and mastectomies have long been considered the biggest pain culprit after breast cancer treatment [142].

However, that conventional belief has been and continues to be challenged, this time by a very large study conducted in Denmark, a country that unlike the United States has a nationalized health care database. The conclusions were reported in the 2009 November edition of *JAMA*. Every type of therapy was a pain culprit, although chemotherapy was not an independent risk factor, and aromatase inhibitors, known to induce muscular and joint pain, were not studied. Out of the 3,257 women who returned the questionnaire, 47% reported some type of pain after an average of two years, and 13% reported it as severe. Young age (below 39), radiation, and ALNDs were the biggest offenders, particularly if they were combined. The overall pain incidence was similar between breast-conservation surgery and mastectomies. Mastectomy patients experienced more "sensory" disturbances, and if they lost a lot of lymph nodes (had ALNDs), the likelihood of *intense* pain increased. On the other hand, the lowest incidence (40%) of *overall* pain was experienced by women over 60 who chose breast-conservation surgery, and by women who bypassed radiation. The only women who did not receive radiation underwent mastectomies and had negative lymph nodes [59].

That comprehensive study provides information and raises questions. Pain from reconstructions was not studied. Although, a 5-year study conducted in Japan found that, when nipple sparing mastectomies with immediate reconstruction were compared to breast-conservation surgeries, the pain frequency was similar [160]. Double mastectomies were not included, thus it is difficult to determine how the choice affects pain outcomes. Some experts have theorized that by definition double mastectomies (CPM) would double pain [88]. Studies comparing different surgeries against CPM, from a pain perspective, would clarify if pain is lowered when radiation or other therapies are avoided, or if the incidence increases. Pain management suggestions are not part of the Denmark study, but the researchers propose that post-breast-therapy pain needs more research, as others have suggested [142,153].

The conclusion that pain occurs with treatments other than mastectomies was noted long before this study. Hence, many no longer refer to pain after breast cancer as *post mastectomy pain syndrome* or PMPS. Instead they use a more encompassing term: *post breast therapy pain syndrome*, or PBTPS [142].

Those of you who have already experienced pain know that icing and heat can be helpful, although both should be used with caution. Icing right before stretching can lead to injury by tightening muscles; therefore, it might be more appropriate afterwards. From one of my last massage therapists, I learned about the biggest mistake people make with ice: they leave it on too long, beyond 15 minutes. Prolonged icing can tighten muscles, once the anti-inflammatory effect has been achieved. In my experience, muscular pain can be diminished by ice if there is swelling and by heat if there is tightness. On the other hand, ice seems to lessen nerve pain and heat might increase it. Relief or increased discomfort can guide you, but be careful in areas of diminished sensation. Most nights I put a gel ice pack in a soft sock before going to sleep. Covering an ice pack for short-term use also diminishes the likelihood of an ice burn in areas of limited sensation. Ice can lessen headaches, ease cervical compression pain, and lower hot flashes, particularly if applied to the forehead, or to the back of the neck. Once the ice pack warms up a little, removing it from its pouch prolongs use.

Aside from ice, other sleep habits made a difference. An adjustable mattress (or memory foam top) minimized my muscular pain. A pillow with good support, but not so thick that it hyperextends the neck, still lessens cervical compression discomfort. Back sleeping is preferred. According to my chiropractor sleeping on the affected side can aggravate upper-torso dysfunctions, particularly if neck, shoulder, or chest muscles have shortened.

Through trial and error I got to know my trigger points and I learned what to do. For hard to reach areas I invested in a good electric massager. Ultrasound light therapy helped for the intense trapezius pain, but it was less effective when that muscle began to relax. Some experts discourage light and heat in proximity to cancer locations; fortunately mine was on the opposite side. Aggressive stretches, such as pulling the front and the back of my arms through overreaching, or from any movements that opened the chest area were needed several times a day. Moist heat or a Jacuzzi helped to relax my muscles, and movement in water was often easier. The interventions in this paragraph were only possible when my nerves regenerated enough to tolerate them. Strengthening efforts also lessened my muscular pain, but I will discuss those in the next section.

Nerve healing and muscular imbalances can interfere with each other. Nerves need rest, time, and lack of barriers to regenerate, while muscles need stretching, and strengthening efforts. Unfortunately nerve deficits often limit muscular movement, potentially for a prolonged period of time. On the other hand, if aggressive muscular strengthening is attempted before sufficient nerve regeneration has taken place, nerve pain might be exacerbated. Many of us are probably experiencing difficulties from this symbiotic duo, and yet I found no resources that could help. The lack of suggestions, when both problems are present, is why the information that combines them is based on personal experience.

If I could turn back the clock, the main thing I would change (particularly during the six weeks of physical therapy) is to have incorporated massage therapy at an earlier stage. Initially I stayed away from massages because I could not lie on my stomach, but I've since learned that mastectomy tables (or pillows) are available in some facilities. Massages might have kept my muscles from getting so out of balance while my nerves were healing.

A good massage therapist, who is familiar with muscular anatomy and pain syndromes, is invaluable. Shortened muscles need to be lengthened in the natural direction of the muscle fibers involved, and tight muscles might release their grip when the right trigger points are massaged.

Other than the different state to state licensure requirements, different levels of training are available to massage therapists. Some obtain a national certification, while others seek training in specialized techniques. For massage therapists interested in adding a marketable certification to their résumé, while increasing their cancer massage knowledge, there are basic, affordable certifications online, including some for breast cancer patients. The Society for Oncology Massages at www.s4om.org has a listing of practitioners with such certifications.

Massage therapy is becoming a respected approach in cancer circles. A search for *oncology massages* generates more information than was available just a couple of years ago. The medical documentation, though rare, can be found for massage therapy to relieve scar tissue from breast-conservation surgery and radiation [38]. ART (at activerelease.com) is usually used for exercise-related injuries and the scar tissue that can result, and yet, massaging scarred tissue to relieve muscular (*myofascial*) pain is suggested in some medical literature [102].

In my opinion, massage organizations are right; massages can lower pain, increase quality of life, and save health care dollars. If the technique becomes an insurance-covered treatment with more insurance carriers, massages might prevent (or lessen) injury and diminish pharmaceutical use. They are constantly lobbying, though so far with limited results. This could be an area of interest for those of you who strive for improved breast cancer legislation.

Acupuncture might lower pain after breast cancer [107], and it is one of the most regulated complementary therapies (CAM) in the United States [136]. License requirements vary, although as with any other field, those with additional training might be the most effective. Practitioners who complete three to four academic years at the master's level in an accredited acupuncture program have extensive training. The Accreditation Commission for Acupuncture and Oriental Medicine (ACAOM) provides information on some practitioners with such advanced Diplomate degrees, and on those with other types of training. ACAOM, at http://www.nccaom.org/ is recognized by the United States Department of Education, for the quality of their acupuncture and Oriental medicine training. At http://www.acupuncture.com/statelaws/statelaw.htm you can find state-by-state licensure requirements.

Acupuncture and massages can be expensive, but that can be handled in different ways. If they are done at medical establishments, such as cancer centers, medical offices, or chiropractic offices, select insurance companies cover part of the cost. Insurance companies might request medical need documentation, and a referral might be needed. At those locations, acupuncturists are bound to maintain basic licensure requirements, and massage therapists might have more experience with chronic muscular pain syndromes. Another way to lessen the cost is to use HSA tax-free funds. Through the calendar year ending in 2013, both still qualify. Plan deductibles might need to be met, and it might be important to keep track of the information in case of an audit. Try to use a facility that is fully licensed and is willing to provide appropriate IRS documentation. Clearly IRS guidelines might change as health care reform gets implemented, and when tax-free deductions are reduced.

Another thing I could have attempted, at a much earlier stage, is a new and hopefully up-and-coming technique called *biopuncture*. This atypical treatment eased my extreme neck tightness when nothing else seemed to work. My rehabilitation reached a new level; less neck tension permitted arm strengthening at higher angles. Biopuncture combines acupuncture and subcutaneous injections of mostly botanical and organic ingredients. It has only been around for 20 years and many are rightfully calling for additional studies. For now, it is mostly being used on those of us who did not respond to traditional approaches, and are counting the length of our chronic pain in years rather than in months. Those who are using it in pain-management circles are finding it promising, in part because of the few reported side effects. Dr. Lee Wolfer, M.D., M.S., a Harvard graduate and an integrative orthopedist practicing in the San Francisco Bay area, has become a proponent of this technique. Although she let me know that oncologists are not comfortable with its use in proximity to cancer areas, and that the benefit might be limited without frequent stretches and in the absence of appropriate muscular strengthening. For more information you can visit Dr. Lee Wolfer's website: Drleewolfer.com/regenerative-injection-therapy-rit/.

Mental techniques were my most valuable tool against every type of pain. Do not discard them simply because the concepts are so abstract. Not all experts agree, but some studies have shown that relaxation techniques, stress management, and hypnosis can help manage chronic pain [119]. The same applies to meditation, visualization, acupuncture, and biofeedback [24].

Dealing with nerve and muscular pain syndromes can be difficult, in part because they can occur from surgery, different types of lymph node dissections, radiation, or chemotherapy. They can also be caused by scar tissue, muscular imbalances, from anti-estrogen therapy, or from a combination of therapies. The pain type and location can vary, and then there is the problem that many of us heal with time while others do not. All of those factors highlight the need to pursue additional research, even though doing so would be challenging.

The multiple causes, the different treatments, the lack of definitive answers, and the various outcomes make it clear that all of us, affected by these complications, need to be informed and involved in our therapies. Combining different approaches opened the door for my rehabilitation to begin, though before that could happen I needed to understand why each was needed.

I wish I had a magic wand or a simple answer for your continued discomforts. I do not, no one does. But don't give up. Remember, healing from nerve damage and from muscular imbalances can still happen long after your treatment has been discontinued, but your perseverance and your involvement are necessary.

❧

REHABILITATION SELF- INVOLVEMENT

There are multiple muscles in the upper torso with confusing names. The information can be intimidating and might discourage self-involvement. Try to at least understand which movements trigger pain in a given area by paying attention to movements. You can also compare one side against the other, visually and manually to make sure the right muscles are moving.

Had I done that earlier, I might have suspected nerve disruptions. I would have understood why my strength was diminishing, rather than increasing, and why my muscular pain was increasing instead of diminishing. Armed with that knowledge, I would have focused on gentler range of motion. The pendulum and circular motions, or *Codman's exercises*, I used after six weeks of physical therapy might have been appropriate. *Passive* range of motion could have been another useful approach. In other words, someone else could have moved the arm that could not move well on its own, or I could have moved it with the opposite arm, had that been a possibility.

Initially I kept a *general* area in mind when I tried to strengthen or relax painful muscles, such as the upper back of the arm, chest muscles, areas between shoulder blades, etc. From that process I understood abnormal compensations, muscular tightness locations, and which areas responded to stretches and massages. That worked for a while, but in time I realized that limiting my comprehension could limit my outcome. Rehabilitative information refers to muscles by name, although I defer detailed anatomy lessons to the experts.

Self-care massage books or trigger point literature can help, assuming you are ready to play an active role in your rehabilitation. *The Trigger Point Self Care Manual* provides muscular anatomy visuals and stretching suggestions [52]. *The Frozen Shoulder Workbook* explains causes for upper-body injuries, appropriate anatomy, and physical therapy approaches [40]. Neither was written for breast cancer pain scenarios, but both provide information on how to treat upper-torso muscular dysfunctions. I believe those are common, often unrecognized, long-term issues after breast cancer treatment. The good news is that many of those, along with the resulting scar tissue, can be diminished. It took years, but with self- and professional massages, proper posture, frequent stretches, and with strengthening efforts, most of my trigger points either disappeared or are manageable.

All patients, who have either nerve or muscular pain, should consult a physical therapist, if either they or their medical providers feel they should, but it is important to understand what is causing the problem. My physical therapists were very knowledgeable, but they did not know scar tissue and endocrine problems were interfering. They still made important contributions. My last therapist taught me the importance of keeping my shoulder pressed down and rolled back, and she showed me how to type with less pain. My six-week therapist explained the aberrant muscular compensations and loosened the left upper arm tightness with his massages, even though he lacked breast cancer complication training. From him I understood the importance of concentrating on the muscles I am targeting; to move in a slow, controlled manner; to keep a good posture; and to persevere. Physical therapists with *breast cancer rehabilitation* training are easier to find in a facility that specializes in cancer treatment. Word-of-mouth referrals can help, but in my opinion none should replace research and interviews.

Basic familiarity with insurance-related language, and annual benefit understanding, might be important. Health insurance companies limit the number of manual therapies in a calendar year. As a saving measure chiropractic care, massage therapy, and physical therapy might be combined under that umbrella term. To personalize rehabilitation, you might need to understand how many visits are allowed in each setting. Most insurance companies want physical therapy completion within a few weeks, as well as frequent progress documentation. Unfortunately, if nerve damage is keeping muscles from working as well as they should, quick progress might not be possible.

It would be helpful, although not likely, if insurance companies allowed less-frequent and shorter physical therapy sessions for several months. When several issues need to progress slowly, traditional physical therapy might worsen pain. Before you run out of benefits for the year you can consider a chiropractor willing to take a slow approach, assuming he or she has rehabilitative training. Different progress guidelines usually apply, and a referral is seldom required. With self-involvement to help personalize treatment, and if recommendations are consistently performed at home, gradual, chiropractic care is another option for chronic pain.

With a better understanding of my limitations, I would have avoided weight-bearing, including yoga poses capable of worsening upper-torso tightness. I would have also enrolled in a tai chi class sooner than I did. Tai chi (or similar techniques) can increase balance and strengthen muscles, without upper-body weight-bearing.

Select YMCAs are helping cancer patients regain their lost muscular strength. Different partnerships make the LIVESTRONG Program possible, though in the Tampa Bay area, it is with Moffit Cancer Center [66]. The program sounds very comprehensive; it is for 12 weeks and with no more than six other survivors in a class. Personal need is assessed before starting, and if the interviewer deems it necessary, the instructor to survivor ratio might be one to one. An internet search for "LIVESTRONG at the YMCA" should provide a list of participating locations.

Thriving After Breast Cancer: Essential Healing Exercises for Body and Mind by Ms. Sherry L. Davis, and Ms. Stephanie Gunning, describes a plan for regaining mobility and strength. This book taught me that a strengthening program can be started when range of motion has been achieved, and that severe pain from mobility is *not* desirable [41]. Clear progress guidelines are described, and it seems to be a good resource for women with lymphedema.

Lymphedema is a long-term concern, even for those of us who lose less lymph nodes [104]. The complication is more likely if a lot of lymph nodes are removed, but 5% to 7% of those who have sentinel lymph node biopsies still develop the condition [140]. The National Lymphedema Network at www.lymphnet.org is one resource for lymphedema-related issues. The Lymphology Association of North America (LANA) at http://www.clt-lana.org/ has a national listing of specialists who passed the North American Certification Exam for Lymphedema Therapists.

The likelihood can be diminished. Slow progressive weight lifting might reduce the incidence of lymphedema [140]. Exercising with a well-fitted lymphedema sleeve might be a consideration for anyone at an elevated risk for the condition, or if it is already present. Preventing infections and cuts on the affected arm and listening to early-lymphedema cues from exercise (or from day-to-day activities) before they become permanent can also lessen the odds. Band exercises are sometimes recommended to breast cancer patients, although they should be held loosely, *not* wrapped [2]. The unwanted compression can cause lymphedema.

Since I was concerned about my early, temporary-lymphedema experience, I spoke with a lymphedema specialist. She agreed that my lymphedema episode, the loss of 10 lymph nodes, and my arm weakness are long-term risk factors. She reiterated that strengthening should be done gradually, and that it is important to avoid sudden unnecessary straining. From her I learned to pay close attention to lymphedema symptoms when I fly. If the symptoms recur at any point, I will wear a lymphedema sleeve and work closely with a specialist.

Some bilateral-mastectomy patients are as worried as I am about arm blood pressure readings and lab work from a lymphedema-prevention perspective. It is best to have our blood pressure taken with a *manual,* rather than with a *self-inflating,* cuff to diminish compression. Leg blood pressure readings are the preferred method, although they can seem inaccurate because they are naturally elevated, and unfortunately, not everyone knows how to take them or interpret them properly. Blood pressure readings and lab work should be done on the side that lost the fewest lymph nodes. If blood pressure is usually normal and different offices are frequented, then it might be possible to reserve them for appointments with primary health care providers.

The Breast Cancer Survivor's Fitness Plan by Dr. Carolyn M. Kaelin, M.D., has a certification from the American Council on Exercise. It offers clear muscular anatomy visuals for each type of breast cancer surgery, along with exercises to strengthen those specific muscles. Muscular strengthening suggestions are based on *experienced* deficits [81]. One of these descriptions let me know that my pectoral muscles needed strengthening, once I was able to address them without my shoulder and neck muscles retightening.

As I started to strengthen my pectoral muscles, the nerve sensitivity that still remained on my chest finally resolved. I had already noticed this connection in other areas: *weak muscles seem to increase, or help to perpetuate, topical nerve sensitivity, and strengthening involved and nearby muscles might lessen it.*

In my opinion, the biggest rehabilitation barrier that many of us experience is the unrealistic time expectation from insurance companies, from therapists, and even from ourselves. Preconceived time limits give the sense that improvement will not happen, unless it occurs within a short period of time. That can be a discouraging thing to hear and believe. I got that sense from two physical therapists, from one chiropractor, from a massage therapist, and from a gentleman interviewing me for a rehabilitative program. I learned to read the doubt in their eyes when I said "nerve damage, failed physical therapy, and over a year and a half after a double mastectomy;" I just refused to be treated by anyone who did not believe in my healing potential.

An update should show how self-involvement can improve outcomes, and how our bodies strive to heal over time. Almost two years after closing the journal (nearly four years after the double mastectomy), the back of my left arm regained most of the lost sensation, and all of my nerve pain is gone. The implants feel completely comfortable, and my pectoral muscles are still getting stronger. Aside from writing, these days I am fairly ambidextrous. Bands, free weights, daily stretching, and proper posture are still playing a key role. My scar tissue is well under control with daily self-massages, and hopefully that will diminish how frequently the implants need to be replaced. I still rely on professional massages once a month to keep me moving forward, and to increase my comfort level.

So far, I've regained over half of my previous strength. I can perform front, lateral, and posterior dumbbell curls with 7 1/2 pounds. I can use seven different machines that require simultaneous arm effort. Front seated row with 35 pounds, overhead cross cable with 30 pounds, seated bicep curl with 20 pounds, and the use of a pectoral fly machine with 20 pounds, are some of my miraculous accomplishments. The weakest muscles in my arms, back, and chest were addressed first. I've increased the weight very gradually, with proper posture, and only one machine at a time. The last point is important. Discomfort from a new challenge might not be noticed for days. Obviously my left arm has gotten stronger, although it is still weaker. I compensate by favoring my right arm when necessary, and by constantly testing my left arm capabilities.

I am having trouble moving past this stage, in part because my neck muscles remain somewhat shortened. Part of the problem is that an important *scalene* (neck muscle) trigger point that needs to be released worsens the cervical compression when it is massaged. Although, thanks to frequent icing to the base of my skull, daily neck massages and stretches, the cervical pain has diminished by more than 90%. My faith for continued improvement remains intact—it has to—someday I am going to be a grandmother. As I have done before, I will accept this plateau for a time, and I'll try to progress at a later date. I am still the weakest person at the gym, although undoubtedly the proudest.

The intricate interaction between the lymphatic system, muscles, nerves, tendons, and the endocrine system's role on neuromuscular health might explain the research barriers, and why sometimes no single approach provides relief. If one of those important players is dysfunctional, others might not be able to perform as well as expected. However, if you try to understand and support that balance, you might maximize your healing potential, lower your muscular tension, and increase your muscular strength. You might just provide an optimal environment for your nerves to heal, lessen your chronic pain, minimize your scar tissue, and improve your quality of life.

꧁꧂

Breast Cancer Screening Guidelines & Dense Tissue Concerns

We have all heard the recommendations made by the United States Preventive Services Task Force (USPSTF) in the fall of 2009, but most of us have not heard the other side of this controversial medical issue. Such information is important. Since opinions vary among those in a position to make breast cancer screening recommendations, each of us needs to understand our risk factors and our preferred approach.

Important societies continue to support the previous guidelines. The American Cancer Society (ACS), the American College of Radiology (ACR), The American

Congress of Obstetricians and Gynecologists (ACOG), and The American Medical Association (AMA), have openly recommended that women continue annual mammograms starting at the age of 40. Studies released after the USPTF recommendations continue to show that, even though all of the benefits might not be noticed for a couple of decades, annual mammograms are important [154].

A detailed critique of the 2009 USPSTF screening recommendations is presented in "United States Preventive Services Task Force Screening Mammography Recommendations: Science Ignored," an article published by the *American Journal of Roentgenology* in the fall of 2010. Data is provided to support the main theories: the USPSTF conclusions were based on only 112 studies (since 514 important ones were excluded), and the annual mammogram radiation exposure is half of what was determined by the USPSTF. It was concluded that limiting mammograms could result in the premature loss of 64,889 women, among those who are now in the 30-to-39-year-old category, assuming 65% of them undergo annual mammograms until the age of 84. If every one of those women screens annually, beginning on the year of their 40th birthday, a total of 99,829 women could benefit from an earlier stage diagnosis over the course of their lifetime [69].

It is important to determine the benefits of mammograms for two-thirds of the population. On average, only two-thirds of eligible women undergo annual mammograms [69]. In other words, the choice to not undergo breast cancer screenings, for whatever reason, was always present. Many women have been taking advantage of that option.

And yet missing screenings may not be such a good idea, particularly for African-American women who screen with less frequency. Even though they have a *lower* incidence of breast cancer, some studies indicate they die in disproportionately *higher* numbers. Less insurance coverage and more aggressive breast cancers could be playing a role; although, since African-American women are usually diagnosed at later stages, they might benefit from annual mammograms [23]. Besides, data published in 2011, and gathered by the American Cancer Society and the National Cancer Institute (NCI), found that for the calendar years 2003 to 2007, the incidence of estrogen-receptor-positive breast cancers in African-American women increased annually [85].

Those who oppose annual screenings have several concerns. They are worried that some slow-growing breast cancers are benign, are over diagnosed, and are over treated [48]. Several studies point to that possibility, though it is not yet known *which* breast cancers will become invasive, and which ones will remain unchanged [46]. I represent that dilemma. I had a slow-growing breast cancer, but it was spreading towards lymph nodes.

Manual exams have also elicited concerns; many of the cancers missed by routine mammograms are aggressive and at an advanced stage by the time they are noted on a self-exam. That is undoubtedly true for most women, but not for all. Tatiana's aggressive cancer was found during a self-exam. Her findings prompted mammograms capable of documenting the progression of her cancer, at an earlier stage than mine. I was an exception to the limited self-exam recommendation for a different reason. My cancer was not palpable, but it was diagnosed at an early-stage because I was familiar with my breast tissue.

Finances are also playing a role. Some screening facilities stand to lose money from the additional personnel, training, and equipment that will be required if the breast density disclosure mandate becomes widespread. In some of the states where such information is now required, insurance companies do not have to pay for screenings other than mammograms. Those that do cover sonograms provide insufficient reimbursement for the procedure. When faced with that dilemma, some women will gladly pay out of pocket for additional screenings. Others will not be willing—or able.

Since younger women have more dense tissue, and breast cancer is more common after the age of 50, many have long believed that mammograms hold limited benefit for women below that age. Dense tissue makes mammograms difficult to interpret, and since much of it tends to lessen after menopause, the screening becomes more accurate. All of that makes sense, except as I've already mentioned, a high percentage of breast density is a known breast cancer *risk factor* in medical literature [30,141,164]. Breast cancer is the *most* frequent cancer in younger women, and the only way to monitor dense tissue is through mammograms. Some specialists believe that only 25% of women still have a lot of breast density after the age of 40 [34], while others believe that figure is closer to 50% for women under the age of 50 [14]. Postmenopausal women are not spared screening difficulties—25% to 33% of them still have dense tissue [14,18].

Because of my extensive dense tissue, I might have benefitted from other screenings in previous years. When questioned, the radiologist who read my ultrasound and my medical oncologist agreed that ultrasounds are useful when there is dense tissue or if a mass looks suspicious, but ultrasounds tend to pick up too many benign things. My breast MRI gave an accurate description of the cancer size and hinted at the possibility of spread, which is more than any other test did.

Even though many believe they are being overused, MRIs can help find breast cancers not noticed by mammograms. Unfortunately they too have false positive results, and at least for now, they are too expensive to become routine. Mine was $2,800. Mammograms remain the screenings of choice because some calcifications, which are noted on mammograms, are considered precancerous.

Breast density is not just a risk factor for breast cancer—a high percentage increases the rate of false-negative results (missed cancers) on mammograms [18]. Invasive cancers, which are most likely to spread to the lymph nodes and metastasize, are more common in masses that do not calcify, and those might be missed by mammograms if there is dense tissue [14]. Ultrasounds increase the false-positive rate, but they also find more breast cancers in women with dense tissue [26,141].

Dense tissue could be a consideration for those of you who are contemplating hormone therapy to manage premenopausal or postmenopausal symptoms. The combination of menopause, high breast density, and the use of estrogen (with either progestin or progesterone), might encourage the development of breast cancer [86]. Not surprisingly, premenopausal women who avoid the therapy might lessen their breast cancer risk [21,43]. That is the complete opposite of using hormone therapy to manage perimenopause symptoms, such as I was prescribed, although in my case my family history, weight, and health habits made it less concerning.

Breast cancer experts, from different international societies, recommended that women with a lot of dense tissue start anti-estrogen therapy *before* a breast cancer episode. They defined high risk as being from *either* family history *or* from high breast density. "Women who have density of more than 75% are at 4 to 5 times greater risk for breast cancer than women with the least dense breasts." [33] The expert recommendation highlights the importance of anti-estrogen therapy, if either breast-conservation surgery or a single-sided mastectomy is chosen. The therapy can *reduce* breast density, and therefore the likelihood of hormone-sensitive cancers on remaining breast tissue. The preventive measure will probably not be implemented. Hormone therapies have a lot of side effects. Besides, hormone-receptor-negative (ER-) breast cancers are also possible with high breast density [176], and anti-estrogen therapy cannot prevent those.

The reason for the connection is unclear, but a lot of dense tissue seems to increase the likelihood of a breast cancer recurrence [67,139]. For women with a history of breast cancer, breast-conservation therapy, and radiation, high mammographic density and obesity appear to be independent risk factors for a local recurrence [131]. A study conducted at Kaiser Permanente in Northern California, and published in 2010, indicated that women with a *lot* of dense tissue, and treated with breast-conservation surgery for DCIS (stage 0), not only have an increased risk of breast cancer in the same breast, but also on the opposite breast [67].

Up-to-date breast density legislation information can be found at www. areyoudense.org. The website was created by a grass-roots organization to inform women about their breast cancer risk from "heterogeneous" dense tissue, and about how adding screenings (such as ultrasounds) can increase early-stage breast cancer detection. Nancy M. Cappello, Ph.D., is the founder of Are You Dense, Inc. The inspiration for the project was her stage IIIc breast cancer diagnosis shortly after a normal mammogram, when she was 40-years old.

All breast cancer screenings have limitations. Even though some experts recommend digital mammography [20], ultrasonography [14], or MRIs to screen dense tissue [20], and new techniques are being tested [34,56], no single test or screening combination is foolproof. Every screening can lead to false-positive results and unnecessary biopsies. One inevitable fact remains: many women need to be screened to benefit a few. Among women who begin annual mammograms at the age of forty, 50% will receive at least one false positive result over 10 years that will lead to more testing, and 5% will undergo a biopsy [167]. Women who chose breast-conservation surgery are particularly familiar with the dilemma—they have more false-positive results and undergo more biopsies [84]. The risk vs. benefit dilemma is a constant for those who are in a position to make recommendations, and for those who need to rely on them.

Since most breast cancers develop in women without a genetic predisposition or a strong family history for the disease [112], we can start by getting to know our personal risk factors. Every woman, with or without a history of breast cancer, should determine how their weight, diet, exercise habits, childbearing age, breast-feeding history, alcohol consumption, past and present hormone use, and percent-age of dense tissue might increase their risk. Hereditary factors, such as Eastern European Jewish ancestry, or first-degree relatives diagnosed with breast cancer at an early age, might prompt genetic testing and/or more frequent screenings.

Gladly, information to start creating individual guidelines is starting to emerge. On April 2012, in a unanimous vote, the FDA's Radiological Devices Medical Advisory Board agreed that the use of *automated ultrasound*, along with mammography, can find more breast cancers in women with a lot of breast density, assuming they have *no* history of breast biopsies or surgeries. This ultrasound cannot tell the difference between breast cancer and scar tissue [18]. It is also becoming clear that for women in the 40-to-49 year old category who have had a breast biopsy, have a lot of dense tissue, and a second degree relative with breast cancer, the benefits of mammograms outweigh the risks [167].

It is important to become proactive and educated, although we are also bound to disagree on the right approach. Breast density information can already be requested during mammograms, but while many women will continue to pursue frequent screenings, even at the risk of false-positive results and biopsies, others will not be willing to go that route.

The debate over mammograms for women under the age of 50 was well underway before the United States Preventive Services Task Forces' recommendations, and will very likely continue for a while. New techniques will continue to be tested and experts will still address the challenges of screening dense tissue. The recommendations might vary, but all are made with our best interest in mind. For now, weighing screening risks against benefits, finding breast cancer at a treatable stage, deciding which cancers are harmless, and screening dense tissue before or after a breast cancer episode, is challenging for all parties involved.

⚒⚒⚒

QUALITY OF LIFE DECISIONS

The information I present is not meant to create more gaps, it is intended to help bridge them. I've tried to highlight that we simply have different viewpoints. Just like screening recommendations, the acceptance of complementary approaches, and the management of endocrine issues are influenced by personal beliefs, personal opinions might be swaying surgical recommendations [77], and even breast cancer research conclusions [129]. Our different approaches might be stemming from how each of us defines *quality of life* and *invasive treatments*. Both are, after all, subjective concepts.

As a result of those natural tendencies, women might be getting more information about the negative consequences of mastectomy choices (including double mastectomy preferences), while the opposite might be the case for breast-conservation surgery (BCS) options. "Current legislation mandating that surgeons inform patients of all options for definitive surgical treatment was motivated by concerns that many women were not being adequately informed about BCS. Ironically, our findings suggest that many women are now not being adequately informed about the option of mastectomy." [83]

Our fear of recurrences, the stress associated with additional therapies, and screening accuracy concerns might make it hard to keep our breast tissue, and yet all are important quality of life considerations. We do miss our intact bodies. The surgery is irreversible, additional surgeries might be needed, recurrences are possible, and pain can accompany mastectomies [88], although the same can be said of every surgical choice. Surgical choice should not be the *only* yardstick by which to measure quality of life [83,156].

The history of cancer, including that of breast cancer, as is so eloquently narrated in *The Emperor of All Maladies* by Dr. Siddhartha Mukherjee, M.D., teaches us that overtime, the breast cancer treatment pendulum has swung from radical surgical, chemical, and radiation approaches, to the minimalist ones which are now the norm [116]. Medical history lessons serve as reminders: nothing stays stagnant for long. In our time, the breast cancer treatment pendulum has the potential to find a new middle ground, a place where a potpourri of choices is the norm.

Breast cancer has been teaching us that a one-size-fits-all approach does not work. Different types of cancers respond to different measures, and screening techniques might be more effective if tailored to individual needs. Can we extend those lessons to surgical choices as well? This could be a nice consolation prize, although it is not the prize we all want—an era without breast cancer. Such a breast cancer age of reason has the potential to resemble the Renaissance. Medical knowledge is already available to us all without the proverbial book burnings. Broader choices would widen the opinion gap, but under those circumstances more medical Leonardo da Vincis could emerge.

Yes, it's true; some of my complications could have been avoided with a single mastectomy, but I might still make a splash. Fewer long-term complications from the therapies I avoided, or fewer local recurrences thanks to the aggressive surgery might leave a positive footprint—or not. Either way, my data, along with that of many others, will help future patients make informed decisions as they search for their own quality of life. That is how breast cancer research progresses. My contribution is minimal compared to the multiple sacrifices others made before me, which granted me so many options.

Those decisions were not made blindly. I was not dealing with a deranged opponent intent on imminent destruction. My opponent was the quiet, dedicated type, working behind the scenes, territorial but not yet working on conquering all, although it had not excluded that possibility. I did not choose radiation or chemical warfare as my weapons. In my opinion, those were more invasive than aggressive surgery.

I know. My eviction notice may not have been heeded and we might again inhabit the same space. I am at peace with my options because they were my choices. The same might not apply, if they had been someone else's decisions.

Dr. Alyssa D. Throckmorton M.D., and Dr. Laura J. Esserman M.D., explain the importance of letting patients decide for themselves. "The key to offering a choice is respecting the choices patients make. Some people will choose one path, others a different one. We need to accept that women will have different values and want different choices. Our job should be to make sure patients have the choices, the information, the time, and environment in which to make an informed, value-driven decision." [156] Our decision should be personalized, even though we are overwhelmed. Only we have to deal with the consequences of our choice.

No, we are not always in agreement. Even though many more women are eligible for breast-conservation surgery, on average, 40% are choosing some type of mastectomy as their treatment. Some institutions are seeing the mastectomy rate climb to 60% [97]. Dr. Charles M. Balch, M.D., and Dr. Lisa k. Jacobs, MD., explain that, "Rather than being alarmed by this trend, we should acknowledge that the rising incidence of total mastectomy emanates from technological advances in our care and patient-driven choices." [8]

They are right. Thanks to an army of researchers and practitioners throughout breast cancer's history, some of us can now make choices, which previous generations could not have contemplated. Depending on our surgical choice, our cancer type, and our cancer stage, some of us can avoid specific therapies and screenings. If we qualify, we can choose innovative surgical techniques and reconstruction methods that might deliver better cosmetic outcomes.

Physicians want their breast cancer patients to make rational decisions—the double mastectomy tsunami is not slowing down [88,158]. In order to make informed personalized choices, future breast cancer patients will need to compare the potential benefits and side effects of each surgical choice and every follow-up therapy. "More than ever, physicians must provide their patients with accurate information on the benefits, limitations, and potential risks of both CPM and alternative strategies (surveillance, chemoprevention)." [159] The information should include long-term recurrence statistics, for individual cancer type and stage beyond 5 or 10 years, as those become available. Being in the minority, and having the same overall survival statistics is no consolation to those who face a local breast cancer recurrence, if they determine that different information would have led to different choices.

All of us, who have been touched by breast cancer, as patients or practitioners, can maximize our contribution to its history. A potpourri of surgical choices will ensure additional research for future generations. In fact, they might learn some of the things we are trying to understand. Under what circumstances are nipple-sparing mastectomies safe? Which treatment combinations are less likely to cause long-term complications, including pain? How do different surgical choices compare from a financial perspective? What guidelines can women use to decide which surgical choice fits their personal definition of quality of life? For now, we can agree on some basic premises: screening accuracy, complication prevention, and side effect management need improvement. Future patients and practitioners will benefit from our data, but they will also assess how we handle the opportunity to set the stage for the age of breast cancer treatment enlightenment.

⊱⊰

The Medical Perspective: An Argument for Less Frequent Lawsuits

Medical care in the United States has built-in barriers—I was not carelessly wronged by the medical establishment. Besides, I have just enough medical understanding to know that no therapy, treatment, or drug is without risk. Some patients have negative outcomes, even when those percentages are low.

My understanding of the medical perspective has been enhanced by knowing many physicians. These friendships taught me that most physicians went into medicine because they wanted to help people, not because of the possible financial rewards. That is a good thing. For the most part, their income is much lower than they had anticipated. If doctors were only interested in monetary gain, they would have skipped many years of school by going into a different profession. That would have saved them quite a bit of money on their exorbitant education, and they would have gotten a lot more sleep in the process.

The combination of various issues might soon create a serious health crisis in the United States. The rising cost of medical school loans, and paying for exorbitant malpractice insurance premiums, are making it difficult to practice medicine. A continued compensation decline may also deter the best of the best from choosing medicine in the future, and that should concern all of us. According to the Association of American Colleges, there is bound to be a shortage of 45,000 *primary* care physicians, as well as a combined shortage of 46,000 medical *specialists* and surgeons by the year 2020, due to limited residency training programs and health care improvements, which are allowing people to live longer [1]. When it comes to primary doctors, it is important to consider that their income is much lower, and that is particularly problematic; they are assigned the difficult task of piecing together our complex medical pictures.

Breast cancer information continues to evolve. Much is still unknown. As explained, not all breast cancers calcify or are easily palpable. The technology to diagnose them is simply not perfect, not even when different methods are combined. Not every lesion can be biopsied—that would result in excessive biopsies. There are guidelines, but not perfect ones. And yet, missed breast cancer lawsuits rank second in medical malpractice frequency [69]. The possibility of nerve damage cannot be eliminated, not even with sentinel lymph node biopsies (SLND). Nerves in the axilla are often cut during lymph node removal [169], although nerve damage can also occur from nerve interruptions to the chest area.

Plastic surgeons get a particularly short end of the stick, even though they cannot control how our bodies heal. Asymmetries and the loss of the entire process can happen with any type of reconstruction. Any infection can ruin our hard-earned reconstructive progress, regardless of surgical technique. Capsular contracture and implant migration are additional risks of reconstructing with implants, and tissue-flap reconstructions carry the risk of grafting difficulties and/or muscular weakness at the grafted areas. If we smoke, need chemotherapy, have or have had radiation to the chest area, our reconstructions can suffer.

Complications from other cancer therapies are also unpredictable; diagnosis and treatment challenges are common. Nerve and muscular pain can stem from different causes (or therapies) and the reason is not always obvious. Not everyone benefits from physical therapy, and not every patient in pain responds to pharmaceuticals. Endocrine problems can be subtle and difficult to treat. The diagnosis can be challenging unless the conditions are advanced.

After years of countless conversations with physician friends, and after my recent encounter with our health care system from the perspective of a consumer, I now believe that we the patients have created many problems. We sue too frequently and have unrealistic expectations. If we sue the very people who are trying to heal us, we are not only harming them and their families—we are harming ourselves. By forcing capable doctors into premature retirement many of us are deprived of their unique expertise, and their absence adds to the physician shortage dilemma.

Very few of us consider our health care a financial priority, and yet we all expect top notch care. Medicine is a business. Someone has to pay, although those who are paying are more interested in profiting, which is a conflict of interests by anyone's definition. Insurance companies seek to profit by reducing our doctor's fees, by refusing claims, by turning away potentially expensive patients, by requesting time consuming authorizations, by increasing our deductibles, and our insurance premiums. Instead of our doctors, and without medical training, some of those employees are deciding which treatments we can undergo. When it comes to insurance coverage, *what we pay is what we get*—try to look beyond the monthly premium. And for reasons beyond my understanding, many patients consider their medical bills optional. How can medical establishments function without getting paid?

We would not sue our neighbor if our child fell on their driveway—neighborhood morale would suffer. And yet, that is what happens when we sue those who are trying to help us heal. Many health care providers fear that each patient is a potential lawsuit capable of taking away their livelihood, which can jeopardize their family's future. That environment discourages out-of-the-box, creative ideas. Going outside safe margins increases the likelihood of a lawsuit. The understandable caution leaves limited options for those of us who are not benefiting from traditional approaches, or if we are not interested in invasive options.

Most people accused of an offense in our legal system are considered innocent until proven guilty, a premise that does not always apply to physicians. In many instances they are considered guilty in *advance*. The challenge is to prove their innocence to a jury with limited medical knowledge, a jury that is far more likely to sympathize with the accuser.

Clearly there are cases of medical negligence that should have a lawsuit. I am not talking about those. I am talking about the unfair ones, which are perhaps the majority. A few years ago my husband was involved in a lawsuit. The suing attorneys wanted him to settle out of court for a "limited settlement," even though he was considered innocent by medical experts. He refused. He wanted to clear his name. That decision resulted in a drawn-out ordeal. It generated intimidating letters, phone calls, and depositions for almost two years, as well as a great deal of unnecessary stress. The lawsuit was eventually dropped. It became clear that he would not be intimidated. His reputation was protected, but two years of attorney's fees raised his group's malpractice insurance premiums.

Another tale merits mentioning. A lawsuit against a physician who became terminally ill during the legal process, except this story has a different ending.

He died before his trial date. On the funeral day his widow was presented with papers indicating the lawsuit would continue against the family's inheritance.

A dear friend was already familiar with the process. He too was also able to clear his name, but he did not think he could endure the lengthy, humiliating process again. When he was presented with yet another lawsuit he committed suicide within the week. We found out much too late that he never came in contact with the person suing him—he was only overseeing the health care provider who did. Those of us who knew him were shocked. He was a very conscientious physician, and one of the kindest men to ever walk on this earth.

Depression and suicide are inherent risks of practicing medicine. The incidence of both is higher for physicians than for professionals in other fields. According to doctorswithdepression.org approximately 300 to 400 physicians commit suicide every year. Those alarming statistics inspired a PBS documentary: *Struggling in Silence*. The title applies. If they seek help for their depression, physicians fear their reputation as medical professionals would be damaged.

Unnecessary lawsuits not only destroy lives and end careers. To keep up with increased malpractice insurance premiums (and low reimbursements), more and more patients need to be seen in a shorter period of time. Unfortunately health care providers are in a time crunch. Their work hours are long and already filled with multiple incidentals. Our present health care system limits the time our health care practitioners have to do extensive research beyond individual specialties, or for patients within their practice. Besides, insurance companies would never reimburse them for such efforts.

It is not an us-versus-them situation, as both sides are interested in improving the system, but things will not change until we are all willing to be part of the solution. We can start by transferring (and keeping) a copy of our medical records—due to electronic incompatibilities most medical offices are unable to share patient information electronically. Some medical records can be transferred between medical establishments, including hospitals, personally, by fax, or by courier with a release form. To help our health care providers understand what might be wrong with us, we should pay close attention to our symptoms. We can be more responsible with our health care dollars, understand that medical professionals cannot heal everything, and that healing takes time. We should follow recommended lifestyle changes, and since no treatment is without risk, we need to become informed and choose our options carefully. If we have a negative experience, we should have an honest dialogue with our medical team.

Most of all, we need to look beyond the immediate monetary gain. It might be hard to change the status quo, and contain health care costs in the United States, unless medical malpractice expenses are addressed. Without tort reform (laws that limit, or cap, the amount of money that patients can receive from a malpractice lawsuit), health care providers will need to continue practicing defensive medicine, and their malpractice insurance premiums will continue to skyrocket. Those issues, along with even lower reimbursements from the Affordable Care Act, will make it difficult for medical establishments to make ends meet.

Health care providers are simply human beings trying to help their patients under continually dwindling resources. They are not God. They face shrinking budgets, constantly changing information, they typically lack in-depth patient histories, and their patient loads are becoming more and more overwhelming. They have incessant legal stressors while having less and less ability to decide what is right for their patients. The situation, including physician shortages, is bound to worsen with health care reform, unless some of these issues are addressed [1]. By doing our part, and by understanding the barriers they face daily, we can help our health care providers deliver the care they want to provide.

⚬⚭⚬

The Sisterhood

An invisible yet golden thread binds all of us breast cancer survivors together. It is a difficult bond to understand unless you are one of us, but perhaps these personal experiences will clarify our sense of connection.

When other survivors reach out, you feel less alone. If you have, or have had breast cancer, you worry about your daughter, your mother, and your sister; you have unwillingly put them at risk. You dare to hope, when a long-time member of the sisterhood reassures you at your first oncology appointment. If your friend is given a breast cancer diagnosis your pain resurfaces, and even though you wish you could keep her from it, you know that you can't. When your daughter goes to a fallen sister's funeral, and you can't be with her because you too had breast cancer, it doesn't seem right. As a complete stranger hugs you at your son's graduation, and shares that the struggle is totally worth it for days such as that one, you know you've been hugged by a sister. After your estranged cousin shares she too has breast cancer a bond is rekindled, then you wonder about an unknown familial connection. Yes, you may shed a tear when a celebrity is diagnosed with breast cancer—she too is now your sister. When your friend dies of breast cancer you cry for yourself, you cry for her loss, you cry for her husband's loss, as well as her children's, but it doesn't take long to realize it could have been your family's loss. If your friend fears her uninsured sister has breast cancer you see the great social divide; you know her care would suffer. When the children of the nonsurvivors walk into your kitchen, the pain in their eyes neither makes sense nor seems fair. As you walk into a room filled with hundreds of breast cancer survivors who are trying to learn how to stay alive for as long as they can it feels overwhelming, then you think epidemic.

✍

EMOTIONAL HEALING

My interest in psychology years ago had an agenda; I believed that if I understood my emotional wounds I would find a way to rise above them. It was a good theory. I did not abuse my children, I learned to avoid risky behaviors, I steered away from abusive relationships, and on the day our first child was born I removed the abusers from our lives. Above all, I adhered to the belief that positive thinking and rational choices, would lead to positive emotions.

It all seemed to work for a while, even though more was brimming underneath; my inability to work because I could not entrust our children to anyone was undeniable, and when our children reached the age of a traumatic event in my childhood I experienced emotional upheavals. I tried therapy, but my sense of control got in the way. The unwelcome emotions from the cancer catharsis showed me how hard it was to keep a semblance of control, and how freeing it was to finally shed it.

If we are unable to verbalize the emotions that cancer elicits, we are more than ill through a significant health crisis: we are emotionally alone. Our family members might get the sense that we neither need them nor want them to be empathetic. Other survivors and professional listeners are important, but unless our loved ones are engaged, we miss the opportunity to mend important relationships. Through our denial, we fail to teach our children the very coping skills that they will eventually need.

Our unwillingness to openly discuss health issues, cancer topics, sexual abuse, pain, and even our mortality extends to society. Sadly, it prevents growth when we need it most. The closed mindedness kept a survivor from posting information about a support group in *The New York Times* as recently as the 1950s, when the publisher refused to print the words *breast cancer* [116]. Many subjects once considered taboo can now be discussed with less discomfort. The evolution continues—I am just doing my part.

Cancer can help us rise above unnecessary biases, shed emotional baggage, and give our suppressed voice an outlet. Try it; it is very freeing. Even though my physical rehabilitation was important and rewarding, the harmony from the generational healing, and the sense of lightness from mourning the abuse transformed me and improved all of my relationships.

Unfortunately I am not alone. According to the U.S. Department of Justice, as many as one-third of girls and one in five boys will be sexually violated in some manner by the time they turn 18. The abuser is typically someone that we know, and it happens in every ethnic, religious, economic, and social circle [32]. I've included these personal aspects, because other cancer survivors might experience similar emotional upheavals.

Dr. Bernie Siegel, M.D., believes that negative influences from our early years, including every type of abuse, sense of loneliness, or feelings of not being loved adequately, tend to create over-pleasing personalities and predispositions to illnesses such as cancer later in life. Cancer patients should find a way to express negative emotions. "When you put your feelings outside, you may heal inside. And you will certainly heal your life, if not your disease." [147] Dr. Siegel is the founder of ECaP (Exceptional Cancer Patients), a nonprofit charitable organization that empowers patients facing cancer and other chronic illnesses. Information about the benefits of mind-body medicine techniques, such as meditation, visualization, and dream interpretation, among other things, can be found at www. ecap-online.org.

We have to perform several balancing acts through our cancer experience. Although for the sake of sanity, difficult topics cannot remain the focus, not even at the peak of trying emotions. When I could, since it was not always possible, I attempted to lessen my concerns by placing an emphasis on humor and gratitude. I tried to focus on what I could do rather than what I could not do, what I had accomplished rather than what I had not, what had been gained rather than what had been lost. Try to let the multiple kind gestures and uplifting words sink in; *cancer is the perfect opportunity for you to learn to receive as well as you give.*

Even though emotional healing after cancer is a personal experience, the fear of a recurrence is our common thread. Ignoring our mortality was much easier to do before cancer, whether we discuss it with our loved ones or not. Several survivors have shared how difficult it is, even years later, when family members refuse to discuss the topic. They feel disconnected and at times resentful towards their well-meaning loved ones. Our mortality awareness can have upsides. We are reminded of how important it is to find joy on a daily basis. We might say *I love you* more often, hug with greater frequency, and it can make sunsets and rainbows more colorful. Those are not permanent states of mind, but we can take occasional glimpses, if we stay open to those possibilities.

Dr. Susan Northrup, M.D., explains why suppressing our voice can be problematic. "There are dozens of studies on breast cancer alone showing that feelings of powerlessness in important relationships and an inability to express the full range of emotions raise the risk of developing breast cancer and lower survival rates from it." [127] In retrospect, I started journaling because I needed to give my often-unwelcome voice an outlet. My willingness to shout it from rooftops for the potential benefit of others means I will no longer suppress it.

Since I wanted to show how breast cancer affects family members, I should probably provide an update on this area as well. In our household cancer discussions, mortality issues, and sexual abuse are not off-limit topics—we are just as likely to discuss them as we are to share a humorous internet video. Neil is thriving as a college student. He is a bright, focused, sensitive young man who can express his feelings with greater ease. We could not be prouder. I accomplished my main parenting goal; I was present when my youngest child graduated from high school. Nicole and her friend Katie dedicated their college essays to how their mother's breast cancer affected their young lives. Despite cancer's imprint, both graduated at the top of their high school class with honors. They are at their first-choice university as college roommates—her mother would have been so proud. These three young adults share one common hope for their future, even though they will be pursuing very different dreams. They hope by the time their generation needs them, dense tissue screening guidelines will be clearer than they were for their mothers. The relationship between my mother and me has blossomed with a wide-reaching, benign ripple effect—a dream come true. My marriage is better than ever. Sandy knows that without his prolonged assistance my healing potential would have been limited, and my financial situation catastrophic. He enthusiastically supports my wish to encourage self-advocacy and participatory medicine. These days he is more willing to contemplate integrative approaches, when traditional medical answers are limited, or if the risks are bound to outweigh the benefit.

Energy medicine is not for everyone, the potential benefits have not been proven by traditional medical standards. However, the World Health Organization acknowledged that acupuncture might help manage over 30 health conditions: asthma, poor memory, menopausal symptoms, fatigue, and various types of pain, including nerve pain, just to name a few conditions.

Some practitioners are open to the possible benefits. In *Energy Medicine for Women* by Ms. Donna Eden, & Dr. David Feinstein, Ph.D., Dr. Susan Northrup, M.D., states, "I have always recognized the importance of energy medicine in my practice. I intuitively understood the influence of my patients' thoughts, fears, desires, relationships, family history, jobs, diet, use of exercise, and overall life-style on their body's energies and the powerful impact of those energies on their health and their illnesses." [44] She also believes that mother-daughter relationships are very important, which is why she dedicated a book to that very topic.

An undisputable connection between childhood abuse and cancer lacks definitive medical evidence, but a higher association has been noted [50,147]. Those of us who intuitively know there is something to it need no such validation. Just like we did not need a study to convince us that sexually abused children can develop high cortisol levels comparable to those of traumatized Vietnam veterans, which are bound to drop during teen years and remain that way well into adulthood. We could have guessed that such long-term cortisol deficiencies can cause predispositions to physical and psychological problems [135], although it is still nice to have the recognition.

Regardless of how or why it is done, the need to explore emotions after a cancer diagnosis is very real—for patients and for families. That is why a branch of psychology has been dedicated to that very purpose, and why it is called psycho-oncology.

⌘

FAITH

If there was an actual choosing of who had to go through this experience and document the evolution, then I was a good choice. My children were at the perfect age: they were old enough to not physically need me so much, and old enough to lend a helping hand and learn from the experience. My marriage was strong. I have a tremendous support system that assisted me during my temporary disability. Finances were not an issue and I did not need to work. The luxury of time allowed me to research, write, and ponder the best rehabilitative approach. I could decipher medical lingo, and I had a sense of exercise physiology. I was an avid reader, and my years as an intensive care nurse taught me how to solve a medical riddle. Thanks to my medical exposure I understood the importance of traditional methods, and my physician husband kept me aware of medical sensitivities. I already had an interest in theology, psychology, an open mind about the power of faith, and about the possible benefits of complementary medicine. And yet, one thing was overlooked by those who set me on this path: I should have been a better typist.

I documented each step of this experience because I *had to*. Something was insisting. The urgency would not be ignored. I tried to stop on more than one occasion. Typing and researching slowed down my rehabilitation by adding pain, but I could not stop. The project kept calling me, telling me that the story needed to be finished, that it might help someone else, and so I persevered, listened to my instincts, and I let faith guide the way. Even now, as I put the finishing touches on these pages, I still have no idea what will become of them, but finish them I must, and trying to share them for the benefit of others will also follow. That is what I must do. Without that altruistic angle I would not be where I am today. It kept me trying to solve my riddle, even when I was ready to give up. If I quit, I would not just be letting myself down, I would be letting others down.

The unusual process has felt very spiritual. Since I felt truly guided, each conquered milestone filled me with gratitude. Faith encouraged me to keep trying. When I allowed doubt to seep in, I felt lonely and lost. This is the biggest leap of faith I have ever taken. I do not know, and have never known, how the process would unfold. But I do know this: without that spiritual dimension, and that sense of purpose, my situation would have felt overwhelming. I would have stopped looking for answers a long time ago.

Many healthcare practitioners do not reinforce the importance of incorporating spirituality into the healing experience, even though the benefits have been documented in breast cancer psycho-oncology literature [58]. Perhaps they fear that a deep sense of spirituality will cause patients to turn down necessary care, or they are not sure if spirituality can enhance medical outcomes, although a few brave souls have begged to disagree.

Dr. Herbert Benson, M.D., Director Emeritus of the Benson-Henry Institute (BHI) and Mind/Body Medical Institute, as well as Associate Professor of Medicine at Harvard Medical School, is perhaps the most iconic of them all. In

Timeless Healing, Dr. Benson describes his controlled observations on meditation. "Whatever your beliefs, when you elicit the relaxation response, you'll be flexing a mind/body mechanism that has proven physiologic merit as well." The relaxation response can elicit in patients a sense of spirituality and even cause spiritual experiences, although he cautions the latter should not be the goal: spiritual experiences do not always occur. Dr. Benson is not afraid to admit that he sometimes acts on instinct, and that instinct can be intertwined with spirituality [13].

Dr. Jeremy Geffen, M.D., shares a similar sentiment: "Although consciously allowing your awareness to abide in the realm of spirit on a regular basis is not a guarantee that physical healing will occur, I deeply believe that it improves the chances, perhaps significantly." [60]

The idea of finding a sense of purpose through adversity has been voiced by others. In *Man's Search for Meaning*, Dr. Victor Frankl, a WWII Nazi concentration camp survivor, theorized that suffering is far more tolerable if we can attach meaning to the experience [55]. His Holiness the Dalai Lama recognizes that, "reflecting on your suffering can reduce your arrogance ... When you are aware of your pain and suffering, it helps you to develop your capacity for empathy." [72] That lesson was well ingrained on Dr. David Biro, M.D. In *Listening to Pain: Finding Words, Compassion and Relief*, he tries to explain the isolating sensation of pain through the use of metaphor in literature. The book's inspiration was Dr. Biro's temporary pain experience, which made him a more compassionate doctor [15].

If you are open to the possibility, cancer can lead you towards spiritual trails, either for the first time or more in depth. This is the *most* important concept I would like to convey to those of you who have been given a cancer diagnosis, regardless of your approach. A nearly palpable sense of spirituality was without question *the* most amazing "gift" that cancer brought my way. I will continue cultivating it and being grateful for it, even though I won't be nearly as grateful for some of the other "gifts." Albert Einstein once said that, "There are two ways to live your life. One is as though nothing is a miracle. The other is as though everything is a miracle." For me, the preferred choice between those two mindsets has never been clearer.

❦

CLOSING STATEMENT

I hope to encourage those of you who are searching for answers to get more involved in your care. Your out-of-the box creative ideas might help you find complication reprieves. *Accept the diagnosis, not the prognosis.* I would also like to help create a voice for those of you who continue to experience difficulties, long after your breast cancer treatment is complete.

I'm not sure why I was able to recuperate as well as I did. I had every symptom that should have been permanent. Perhaps the nerve in question was not completely severed. Undergoing only surgical treatment might have allowed my body to heal better than it could have otherwise, although breaking up the scar tissue and rehabilitating in a gradual, sequential manner might have also been instrumental. Believing that my body had the capacity to heal if I supported it properly and gave it time could have played a role, and the same applies to the resolution of my endocrine issues. If that was the case, then unrecognized endocrine imbalances might be keeping other survivors fatigued and in pain.

My grandmother used to tell us that we should pray as though everything depends on God, but work as though nothing does. I have tried to do just that. I have combined faith with effort in my rehabilitation experience, in the documentation of my journey, with the introspection and research that were required to write it, and in my wish to help others by sharing my story as clearly and as truthfully as possible.

Regardless of what becomes of my writing, it already helped me heal in every way possible, including physically. These days I inhabit my body with an almost forgotten sense of harmony. At times I barely recognize it as my own. My mornings are always off to a good start when I wake up with my arms painlessly positioned behind my head. On those occasions, and when I perform simple tasks, I stop to recognize how miraculous it is to move without pain. I am even jogging on a regular basis with an indescribable sense of joy. Knowing that I have the pain-free energy to do that does feel like I finally stepped off my pain trail, and like I'm actually flying.

☙❧

ACKNOWLEDGEMENTS

The various survivors who so candidly shared their experience and concerns, and even those who are suffering in silence, deserve the first acknowledgement; you have been my motivation and inspiration. To my surgical oncologist, your impressive résumé pales by comparison to your humanity—you are a surgical Leonardo da Vinci. I need to thank my plastic surgeon for allowing so much involvement, for believing in this project, and for my superior cosmetic outcome. To both of my integrative physicians, thank you for making such important contributions; I understand why you practice integrative medicine. Dr. Minton, M.D., my medical oncologist, your reputation is well deserved. My Body Talk therapist, Dr. Gloria Payne, Ph.D., thanks for opening Pandora's box—I have never felt lighter. I want to thank my pain specialist for identifying the cause of my pain; you will be the first person I call when I am ready for a nerve block. Dr. Fox, M.D, my asthma specialist for the past 15 years, you embody the best of what participatory medicine can be. I've tried to emulate our medical relationship in other aspects of my care. Dr. E. Harris, M.D., and Dr. T. Cardoso, M.D., thanks for your assistance above and beyond the call of friendship. To my physical therapist of six weeks, I am sorry my body was not ready for your wisdom, but I know it is vast. I hear you now, every time I do what you so expertly taught me, I am finally ready. Andrew Harden, my ART massage therapist, you have magic hands, even if you are not prepared to admit it. Anisha and Dr. Dziubinski, (my acupuncturists), I don't know how you do what you do but I am glad that you do it. Kim Motissi, Heather Houston, and Dr. Jeffrey T. Farrell, my last massage therapists and chiropractor, thank you for putting the finishing touches on what others had already started. To every receptionist, volunteer, medical records attendant, pathologist, radiologist, and technician who crossed my path, your contributions are the sprockets that keep the wheels of oncology moving forward. Ravin Sajnani, thanks for the many hours you spent retrieving articles from the medical library. Ruth Goodman, outstanding proofreading and personal touch are an unbeatable combination. Katherine, my medical editor, Diane Ricardi and Molly Byock, yet two other writing advisors, I would have been lost without your valuable input. Debbi Stocco, my cover and interior page designer, your patience and creativity are evident in every single page.

Mom, if our reconnection had been the only positive outcome from this experience, then it would have been worth it. I see you. Edith, I have consistently found love and acceptance in your loving family "huppa" for nearly 26 years. Cielo, your unconditional love constancy has not gone unnoticed. Ruby, thanks for teaching me the true meaning of the word "resilience," and for letting me into your loving inner circle. Sandy, we may be cut from different cloths, but together we make a beautiful tapestry. We don't always walk the same trails, but they always lead us back to each other's heart. Neil and Nicole, for you I have tried to become my best self. I thought I gave birth to you, but on the contrary, it was you who gave birth to me. Andrew, my stepson, you have never been afraid to walk your own trails (quite literally!). Thanks for setting a good example and for the cover photo contribution. My siblings and extended family, you are ensuring that love and respect become our children's most valuable inheritance. Tatiana, we have been in the trenches of laughter and tears about our ordeals on more occasions than either of us can recall. You have validated my experience; I hope I have served you as well. To the many young adults, who have graced our home with their presence, thank you for letting us into your hearts. I am hopeful about the future—your minds are already open to endless possibilities. Magic, our canine family member, thank you for reminding me of the most important things in life: appreciate the ones you love, make the most of your morsels while remaining hopeful for more, and always walk your own trails. Finally and without parallel, the most important acknowledgement goes to the powers that be, for setting me on this path. Thank you for letting me take a glimpse at the brilliant colors that can only be found in spiritual trails.

⊗∅©

References & Related Reading

1. *AAMC: Tomorrow's Doctors, Tomorrow's Cures.* "Physician Shortages to Worsen Without Increase in Residency Training." www.aamc.org Source: AAMC Center for Workforce Studies, June 2010 Analysis. Accessed 5/2/2011.

2. Aaronson, Naomi. *"Exercise: When at Lymphedema Risk After Breast Cancer."* http://www.recovercisesforwellness.com/lymphedema.htm Accessed 1/7/2013.

3. Abel, EK. Subramanian SK. *After the Cure: the Untold Stories of Breast Cancer Survivors.* New York & London: New York University Press. 2008. [Chronic fatigue and cognitive impairments, from chemotherapy and radiation, were the most frequent and disruptive symptoms. A few survivors found complementary therapies beneficial but unaffordable without insurance recognition, while others were hesitant because they were not endorsed by health care providers. Since complications were not always acknowledged by medical teams, some women could not receive disability benefits. Others had less disabling symptoms but were still forced to change careers. Dr. Patricia Ganz, M.D., advocates for more research, even though the various symptoms would be difficult to measure. Book overview]. [There are 2.5 million breast cancer survivors in the USA. p. 139].

4. Albom, Mitch. *Tuesdays with Morrie: An Old Man, a Young Man, and Life's Greatest Lesson.* New York: Broadway Books. 2002 edition. [When necessary, professor Morrie grieved his impending death for a limited period in the morning, then focused on what was still good in his life for the rest of the day. p. 57].

5. Antonova L, Aronson K, Mueller CR. "Stress and Breast Cancer: from Epidemiology to Molecular Biology." *Breast Cancer Research.* 2011. 13:208. Doi: 10.1186/bcr2836. http://breast-cancer-research.com/content/pdf/bcr2836.pdf Accessed 11/11/2011.

6. Arriagada R, Lê MG, Guinebretière JM, Dunant A, et al. "Late Local Recurrences in a Randomized Trial Comparing Conservative Treatment with Total Mastectomy in Early Breast Cancer Patients." *Annals of Oncology.* 2003; 14(11): 1617-1622.

7. Azvolinsky, Anna. "Physical Activity in Cancer Survivors Associated With Better Health Outcomes." *Cancernetwork: home of the journal Oncology.* Summarized from an analysis by the National Cancer Institute (NCI). http://www.cancernetwork.com/breast-cancer/content/article/10165/2069862 Posted 5/9/2012. Accessed 2/6/2013.

8. Balch CM, Jacobs LK. "Mastectomies on the Rise for Breast Cancer: The Tide Is Changing." *Annals of Surgical Oncology: Official Journal of the Society of Surgical Oncology.* Editorial. 2009; 16(10): 2669-2672.

9. Barclay, L. "New Breast Cancer Screening Guidelines Opposed by Societies." Medscape Medical News. Summarized from *Annals of Internal Medicine.* 11/17/2009. 2009; 151: 716-726,727-737,750-752. Posted 11/19/2009. http://www.medscape.com/viewarticle/712720 Accessed 4/21/2011.

10. Barton, Debra. "Integrative Oncology; Integrative Medicine: Not Just Garnish." *Cancer Network; Home of the Journal Oncology Nurse Edition.* Vol. 26 No. 5. Posted 5/9/2012. http://www.cancernetwork.com/nurses/content/article/10165/2060868 Accessed 5/10/2012.

11. Beadle BM, Woodward WA, Buckholz TA. "The Impact of Age on Outcome in Early-Stage Breast Cancer." *National Institute of Health (NIH), Public Access.* Author Manuscript. PMC3041510. Published in *Seminars in Radiation Oncology.* 2011; 21(1): 26-34. Accessed 1/7/2013.

12. Bedrosian I, Hu C-Y, Chang G J. "Population-Based Study of Contralateral Prophylactic Mastectomy and Survival Outcomes of Breast Cancer Patients." *Journal of the National Cancer Institute (JNCI).* 2010; 102(6): 401-409. DOI: 10.1093/jnci/djq018. *Oxfordjournals.org.* http://jnci.oxfordjournals.org/content/102/6/401 Accessed 11/15/2011.

13. Benson, Herbert. Stark M. *Timeless Healing: The Power and Biology of Belief.* New York, NY: Scribner. 1996. ["Whatever your beliefs, when you elicit the relaxation response, you'll be flexing a mind/body mechanism that has proven physiologic merit as well." p. 168]. [The relaxation response can elicit a sense of spirituality and even cause spiritual experiences, although the latter should not be the goal; spiritual experiences do not always occur. p. 167]. [Dr. Benson admits that he sometimes acts on instinct, and that instinct can be intertwined with spirituality. pp. 195-196].

14. Berg WA, Blume JD, Cormack JB, et al. "Combined Screening with Ultrasound and Mammography vs. Mammography Alone in Women at Elevated Risk of Breast Cancer." *JAMA: Original Contribution.* 2008; 299(18): 2151-2163. Corrections *JAMA* 4/21/2010; 303(15): 1482.

15. Biro, David. *Listening to Pain: Finding Words, Compassion, and Relief.* New York, NY: W.W. Norton & Company, Inc. 2010. ["Studies have shown that the more detailed those descriptions are, the better physicians are at pinpointing the source of pain and administering appropriate treatment." p. 14-15]. [Dr. Biro tries to explain the isolating sensation of pain through the use of metaphor in literature. His temporary pain experience helped him become a more compassionate doctor. Book overview].

16. Block, Keith I. *Life Over Cancer: The Block Center Program for Integrative Cancer Treatment.* New York, NY: Bantam Books. 2009. [Dr. Block counsels those of us who are interested in trying to prevent a recurrence from a variety of perspectives, including nutrition and endocrine balances. Book overview]. [Altered cortisol levels (including chronic low levels), poor sleep, low body weight, and abnormal glucose metabolisms, can create a negative endocrine terrain that might increase the likelihood of a cancer recurrence. pp. 408-428]. [Magnesium can help lower muscular pain and increase exercise tolerance. p. 423].

17. Bokhari F, Sawatzky JAV. "Chronic Neuropathic Pain in Women After Breast Cancer Treatment: The Human Response to Illness Model." Adapted from *Pain Management Nursing*. 2009; 10(4):197-205. Posted *by Med Scape Nurses News*. http://www.medscape.com/viewarticle/715640 DOI: 02/26/2010. Accessed 3/25/2011.

18. Boughton, Barbara. "FDA Panel Votes to Expand Use of Automated Breast Ultrasound." *MedscapeNews Nurses*. Posted: 04/11/2012. Based on an expert advisory committee vote of the US Food and Drug Administration (FDA) on 4/11/2012. http://www.medscape.com/viewarticle/761934 Accessed 5/14/2012.

19. Bowthorpe, Janie A. *Stop the Thyroid Madness: A Patient Revolution Against Decades of Inferior Thyroid Treatment*. Florence, CO: Laughing Grape Publishing. 2008. [It might be necessary to address low cortisol levels in order to increase thyroid replacement doses to proper levels. pp. 70-71]. [In extreme adrenal fatigue, the use of Hydrocortisone might be necessary for months. pp. 105-107].

20. Boyd NF, Guo H, Martin LJ, et al. "Mammographic Density and the Risk and Detection of Breast Cancer." *The New England Journal of Medicine; Original Article.* 2007; 356(3): 227-236.

21. Boyd NF, Melnichouk O, Martin LJ, Hislop G, et al. "Mammographic Density, Response to Hormones, and Breast Cancer Risk." *Journal of Clinical Oncology.* 2011; 29(22): 2985-2992.

22. Boyles, Salynn. "Breast Cancer Treatment Ups Long-Term Survival." *WebMD: Better Information Better Health*. Posted 5/12/2005. http://www.webmd.com/breast-cancer/news/20050512 Accessed 5/18/2011.

23. *Breastcancer.org*. ["Infections After Breast Surgery Costly: US Study." Published 1/21/2008. Accessed 6/27/ 2010. http://www.breastcancer.org/treatment/surgery/new research/20080121b.jsp]. ["Acupuncture." Modified 9/17/2012. Accessed 1/7/2012. http://www.breastcancer.org/treatment/comp_med/types/acupuncture.jsp]. ["Lack of Insurance Affects African Americans' Breast Cancer Prognosis More Than Whites." Modified 11/19/2012. Accessed 12/6/2012. http://www.breastcancer.org/symptoms/new_research/20100625b.jsp].

24. Brenman, Ephraim, editor. "Pain Management Health Center: Pain Management Alternative Therapy." *WebMD: Better information. Better health*. Posted 3/1/2007. Reviewed by doctors at The Cleveland Clinic Center for Integrative Medicine. http://www.webmd.com/pain-management/guide/pain-management-alternative-therapy Accessed 5/20/2012.

25. Brody GS, Long JN, editor. "Silicone Breast Implant Safety and Efficacy." *Medscape Reference: Drugs Diseases & Procedures*. http://emedicine.medscape.com/article/1275451 Updated 4/25/2012. Accessed 7/2/2012.

26. Brice, James. "Ultrasound Adds to Mammography's Diagnostic Power for At-Risk Women." *Medscape Medical News*. Posted 3/12/2012. Summarized from Berg, et al. "Detection of Breast Cancer with Addition of Annual Screening Ultrasound or a Single Screening MRI to Mammography in Women With Elevated Breast Cancer Risk." *JAMA*; Original Contribution. 2012; 307(13):1394-1404. http://www.medscape.com/viewarticle/761459 Accessed 5/12/2012.

27. Bryce J, Bauer M, Hadji P. "Aromatase Inhibitor-Associated Bone Loss." *Medscape Today News*; Oncology Nursing Forum. http://www.medscape.com/viewarticle/743577 2011; 38(3): 273-276.

28. *Cancer.org*. ["Mammograms and Other Breast Imaging Procedures; Diagnostic Mammograms." Revised 7/13/2012. Accessed 1/7/2012]. ["Women's Health and Cancer Rights Act: The Federal Law." Revised 9/18/2012. Accessed 2/11/2013].

29. Caraccio N, Natalie A, Sironi A, et al. "Muscle Metabolism and Exercise Tolerance in Subclinical Hypothyroidism: A Controlled Trial of Levothyroxine." *The Journal of Clinical Oncology & Metabolism*." 2005; 90(7): 4057-4062.

30. Chen JH, Hsu FT, Shi HN, et al. "Does Breast Density Show Difference in Patients with Estrogen Receptor-Positive and Estrogen Receptor-Negative Breast Cancer Measured on MRI?" *Annals of Oncology*. 2009; 20(8): 1447-1449.

31. Cheville AL, Tchou J. "Barriers to Rehabilitation Following Surgery for Primary Breast Cancer." *Journal of Surgical Oncology*. 2007; 95(5): 409-418.

32. *Childhelp.org*. For PARENTS: MYTHS vs. FACTS about child sexual abuse and prevention education. http://www.childhelp.org/page/-/pdfs/MYTHS-FACTS.pdf Accessed 7/19/2011.

33. Chustecka, Zosia. "Experts Call for Greater Use of Breast Cancer Prevention." *Medscape Medical News > Oncology*. Posted 3/30/2011. Summarized from "Preventive Therapy for Breast Cancer: A Consensus Statement." *Lancet Oncology*. 2011; 12(5): 496-503. DOI 3/25/2011. http://www.medscape.com/viewarticle/739920 Accessed 5/3/2011.

34. Chustecka, Zosia. "Molecular Breast Imaging Detects Cancer in Dense Breasts." *Medscape Medical News*. Primary Source: 2008 Washington D.C. Breast Cancer Symposium (BCS); Abstract 68. Presented 8/7/2008. www.medscape.comview-article/580258 Accessed 4/2/2011.

35. Collins DE, Moore CP, Clay KF, et al. "Can Women with Early-Stage Breast Cancer Make an Informed Decision for Mastectomy?" *Journal of Clinical Oncology*. 2009; 27(4): 519-525.

36. Conger, Krista. "Combination Treatment for DCIS Breast Cancer Improves Survival Rates, Scientist Reports." *Stanford School of Medicine*. DOI: 3/11/2011. http://med.stanford.edu/ism/2011/march/wapnir.html Accessed 5/19/2011.

37. Cousins, Norman. *Anatomy of an Illness: As Perceived By the Patient.* New York, NY: W.W. Norton & Company, Inc. 1979. [Individuals with leprosy injure themselves because they cannot feel pain. pp. 99-120]. [Mr. Cousins used participatory medicine, self-advocacy, adrenal support, and humor to lessen stress and heal the adrenal glands. Book overview].

38. Crawford JS, Simpson J, Crawford P. "Myofascial Release Provides Symptomatic Relief from Chest Wall Tenderness Occasionally Seen Following Lumpectomy and Radiation in Breast Cancer Patients." *International Journal of Radiation Oncology: *Biology*Physics.* 1996; 34(5): 1188-1189.

39. Crowe JP, Patrick RJ, Randall RJ, et al. "Nipple-Sparing Mastectomy Update: One Hundred Forty-Nine Procedures and Clinical Outcomes." *Archives of Surgery.* 2008; 143(11):1106-1110.

40. Davies, Clair. *The Frozen Shoulder Workbook: Trigger Point Therapy for Overcoming Pain & Regaining Range Of Motion.* Oakland, CA: New Harbinger Publications Inc. 2006. [Trapezius tightness can explain mid-back pain, shoulder pain, neck pain, as well as headaches. pp. 153-155]. ["Of all the muscles in the body, the trapezius is the one most commonly afflicted with trigger points." p. 153]. [Ms. Clair explains causes for upper-body injuries, appropriate anatomy, partner techniques, and physical therapy approaches. Book overview].

41. Davis, Sherry L. Gunning, Stephanie. *Thriving After Breast Cancer: Essential Healing Exercises for Body and Mind.* New York: Broadway Books. 2002. [A strengthening program can be started when range of motion has been achieved. p. 29]. [Severe pain from mobility is not desirable. p. 49].

42. Dean, Carolyn. *The Magnesium Miracle: Discover the Missing Link to Total Health.* New York: Ballantine Books. 2007. [Supplemental magnesium might improve sleep and reduce migraine headaches. Fatigue syndromes, nerve disorders, and bronchial spasms can be worsened by this deficiency, and poor diet and stressful situations might exasperate it. Book overview].

43. Doheny, Kathleen. "Studies Confirm Link Between Breast Density and Cancer: As Density Drops Over Time so Does Risk, One Study Finds." *HealthDay.* Report from the 2010 Washington D.C. Annual Meeting of the American Association of Cancer Research. http://health.usnews.com/health-news/family-health/cancer/articles/2010/04/21 Posted 04/21/2010. Accessed 4/27/2011.

44. Eden, D. Feinstein, D. *Energy Medicine for Women: Aligning Your Body's Energies to Boost Your Health and Vitality.* U.S. printing in New York, NY: Penguin Group. 2008. ["I have always recognized the importance of energy medicine in my practice. I intuitively understood the influence of my patients' thoughts, fears, desires, relationships, family history, jobs, diet, use of exercise, and overall lifestyle on their body's energies and the powerful impact of those energies on their health and their illnesses." Foreword, *xvii*].

45. Edwards PD, Toppings D, Kontaridis MI, et al. "Arginine-Enhanced Enteral Nutrition Augments the Growth of a Nitric Oxide-Producing Tumor." *Journal of Parenteral and Enteral Nutrition: an International Journal of Nutritional and Metabolic Support.* 1997; 21(4): 215-219.

46. Elmore JG, Fenton JJ. "Ductal Carcinoma In Situ (DCIS): Raising Signposts on an Ill-Marked Treatment Path." *National Cancer Institute (JNCI).* 2012; 104(8): 569-571. DOI:10.1093/jnci/djs184. http://jnci.oxfordjournals.org/content/104/8/569 Published online 4/5/2012. Accessed 5/13/2012.

47. Eremin, Oleg. *L-Arginine: Biological Aspects and Clinical Application.* Georgetown, Texas: R.G. Landes Company. 1997. [L-Arginine might increase cancer cell proliferation through indirect mechanisms. p. 53]. [L-Arginine is a Nitric Oxide precursor. p. 142].

48. Esserman L, Shieh Y, Thompson I. "Rethinking Screening for Breast Cancer and Prostate Cancer." *JAMA.* 2009; 302(15): 1685-1692.

49. Fatouros M, Roukus DH, Arampatzis I, et al. "Factors Increasing Local Recurrence in Breast-Conservation Surgery." *Expert Review of Anticancer Therapy.* 2005; 5(9): 737-745. http://www.expert-reviews.com/doi/abs/10.1586/14737140.5.4.737 DOI: 10.1586/14737140.5.4.737. Accessed 1/7/2013.

50. Felitti VJ, Anda, RF, Nordenberg D, et al. "Relationship of Childhood Abuse and Household Dysfunction to Many of the Leading Causes of Death in Adults: The Adverse Childhood Experiences (ACE) Study." *American Journal of Preventive Medicine.* 1998; 14(4): 245-258.

51. Fernandes-Taylor S, Bloom JR. "Post-Treatment Regret Among Young Breast Cancer Survivors." NIH Public Access Manuscript. PMCID: PMC3015023. http://www.ncbi.nlm.nih.gov/pmc/articles/PMC3015023/ *Psychooncology.* 2011; 20(5): 506-516.

52. Finando, Donna. *Trigger Point Self-Care Manual: For Pain Free Movement.* Rochester, Vermont: Healing Arts Press, a Division of Inner Traditions International. 2005. [The workbook provides muscular anatomy visuals and stretching suggestions. Book overview]. [Trigger points in the trapezius might develop from "overload, compression, and trauma." p. 42]. [The trapezius is the main muscle that supports the weight of the arms. p. 43].

53. Fogoros, Richard N. "Cardiac Effects of Thyroid Disease." *About.com: Heart Health Center.* http://heartdisease.about.com/od/lesscommonheartproblems/a/thyroidheart.htm Updated 11/13/2011. Accessed 1/2/2011.

54. *Fox News.* "More Women Get Both Breasts Removed With Cancer in Only One." Posted 10/23/2007. http://www.foxnews.com/story/0,2933,304239,00.html Accessed 5/18/2011.

55. Frankl, Victor E. *Man's Search for Meaning.* New York, NY: A Washington Square Press Publication. 1984. [Suffering is more tolerable, if we attach meaning to the experience. p. 170].

56. Freiherr, Greg. "Breast CT Scanners Skip Compression, Show Cancer in 3D." Medscape Radiology > Innovations in Radiology. *Medscape Nurses News.* Posted 01/24/2012. http://www.medscape.com/viewarticle/757046?src=nl_topic Accessed 1/26/2012.

57. Frost MH, Slezak JM, Tran NV, et al. "Satisfaction After Contralateral Prophylactic Mastectomy: the Significance of Mastectomy Type, Reconstructive Complications, and Body Appearance." *Journal of Clinical Oncology.* 2005; 23(31): 7849-7856.

58. Gall TL, Cornblat MW. "Breast Cancer Survivors Give Voice: A Qualitative Analysis of Spiritual Factors in Long-Term Adjustment." *Psycho-Oncology.* 2002; 11(6): 524-535.

59. Gärtner R, Jensen M-B, Nielsen J, Ewertz M, Kroman N, Kehlet H. "Prevalence of and Factors Associated With Persistent Pain Following Breast Cancer Surgery." *JAMA.* 2009; 302(18): 1985-1992.

60. Geffen, Jeremy R. *The Journey Through Cancer: Healing and Transforming the Whole Person.* Second edition. New York: Three Rivers Press. 2006. [Up to 80% of cancer patients resort to complementary health care. p. 24]. [In the US more cash is spent on complementary and alternative medicine, than on out-of-pocket medical premiums, including hospitals. p. 23]. [Emotional, spiritual, and social aspects should be considered. We should treat our bodies as a "garden" by adding rest, exercise, massage therapy, nutrition, supplementation, yoga, journaling, visualization, acupuncture, chiropractic care, homeopathy, Reiki, and therapeutic touch. pp. 95-131]. [DHEA might encourage estrogen and testosterone production. p. 115]. ["Although consciously allowing your awareness to abide in the realm of spirit on a regular basis in not a guarantee that physical healing will occur, I deeply believe that it improves the chances, perhaps significantly." p. 225].

61. Geiger AM, West CN, Nekhlyudov L, et al. "Contentment with Quality of Life Among Breast Cancer Survivors With and Without Contralateral Prophylactic Mastectomy." *Journal of Clinical Oncology.* 2006; 24(9): 1350-1356.

62. Giuliano AE, Hunt KK, Ballman KV, et al. "Axillary Dissection vs. No Axillary Dissection in Women with Invasive Breast Cancer and Sentinel Node Metastasis: A Randomized Clinical Trial." *JAMA.* Original contribution. 2011; 305(6): 569-575.

63. Goldflam K, Hunt KK, Gershenwald JE, et al. "Contralateral Prophylactic Mastectomy: Predictors of Significant Histological Findings." *Cancer.* 2004; 101(9): 1977-1986.

64. Goodier, Rob. *Medscape.com.* "Few Women Regret Prophylactic Mastectomy." From *Reuter's Health Information.* Summarized from study presented @ the 2011 American Society of Breast Surgeons' annual meeting in Washington, DC. www.medscape.com/viewaetcle/742111 Posted 5/4/2011. Accessed 5/7/2011.

65. Gradishar, William J. "Ramifications of Breast-Conserving Surgery for Ductal Carcinoma in Situ: Ten-year Follow-Up Shows High Rates of Subsequent Invasive Procedures." Journal Watch Women's Health. 4/26/2012. http://women-shealth.jwatch.org/cgi/content/full/2012/426/6 Accessed 5/13/2012.

66. Green, Susan. "Cancer Survivors turn to YMCA: The Livestrong at the Y Program Offers Workouts and Motivation." *The St. Petersburg Times*. Published Apr. 8th 2011.

67. Habel LA, Capra AM, Achacoso NS, Janga A, Acton L, et al. "Mammographic Density and Risk of Second Breast Cancer after Ductal Carcinoma *In Situ*." *Cancer Epidemiology, Biomarkers & Prevention*. 2010; 19(10): 2488-2495.

68. Harpham, Wendy S. *When a Parent Has Cancer: A Guide to Caring for Your Children*. Second Edition. New York, NY: Harper Collins. 2004.

69. Hendrick ER, Helvie MA. "United States Preventive Services Task Force Screening Mammography Recommendations: Science Ignored." *American Journal of Roentgenology: Diagnostic Imaging and Related Sciences:* web exclusive. 2011; 196(2): W112-W116. http://www.ajronline.org/content/196/2/W112.full DOI:10.2214/AJR.10.5609. Accessed 3/18/2011.

70. Herrington LJ, Barlow WE, Yu O, et al. "Efficacy of Prophylactic Mastectomy in Women with Unilateral Breast Cancer: A Cancer Research Network Project." *Journal of Clinical Oncology*. 2005; 23(19): 4275-4286.

71. Hinrichs CS, Watroba NL, Rezaishiraz H, et al. "Lymphedema Secondary to Post Mastectomy Radiation: Incidence and Risk Factors." *Ann. Surg. Oncology*. 2004; 11(6): 573-80.

72. His Holiness the Dalai Lama, Cutler, Howard C. *The Art of Happiness: A Handbook for Living*. New York: Penguin Group. 1998. [Difficult situations and emotions are simply part of life, the difference lies in how we respond. pp. 150-152]. ["Reflecting on your suffering can reduce your arrogance... When you are aware of your pain and suffering, it helps you to develop your capacity for empathy." p. 206].

73. Hollifield M, Sinclair-Lian N, Warner TD, et al. "Acupuncture for Posttraumatic Stress Disorder: A Randomized Controlled Pilot Trial." *Journal of Nervous and Mental Disease*. 2007; 195(6): 504-513.

74. Houssami N, Abraham LA, Miglioretti DL, et al. "Accuracy and Outcomes of Screening Mammography in Women with a Personal History of Early-Stage Breast Cancer." *JAMA*. 2011; 305(8): 790-799.

75. Jacobs, Bradley MD. MPH. "East Meets West: Integrating Complementary Medicine into Your Care." *Cancer Supportive Survivorship Care*. www.cancer-supportivecare.com/eastwest.html Updated 4/25/2011. Accessed 5/21/2012.

76. Johnson, Kathy. "'Chemo Brain' May Actually Be Worry and Fatigue, Says Study." *Medscape Medical News*. Summarized from abstract S6-3. Presented @ the 35th Annual San Antonio Breast Cancer Symposium (SABC) on 12/7/2012 by Dr. Bernadine Cimprich. http://www.medscape.com/viewarticle/775895 Accessed 1/30/2013.

77. Jones NB, Wilson J, Kotur L, et al. "Contralateral Prophylactic Mastectomy for Unilateral Breast Cancer: An Increasing Trend at a Single Institution." *Annals of Surgical Oncology*. 2009; 16(10): 2691-2696.

78. Jung BF, Ahrendt GM, Oaklander AL, et al. "Neuropathic Pain Following Breast Cancer Surgery: Proposed Classification and Research Update." *Pain*. 2003; 104(1-2): 1-13.

79. Jung, Carl G. *Man and his Symbols*. Garden City, New York: A Windfall Book. 1964. [Dr. Jung spent years gathering information from different cultures and religious philosophies. Archetypal symbols can reveal themselves in dreams, feelings, or with intuition that can seem life changing. pp. 58-82 & p. 304].

80. Jung, CG. Campbell, Joseph, editor. *The Portable Jung*. New York, NY: The Viking Press Inc. 1971. [Dr. Jung walked away from the opportunity to work with Sigmund Freud in 1913 after a symbolic dream. Chronology *xxv*].

81. Kaelin, Carolyn M. *The Breast Cancer Survivor Fitness Plan: Reclaim Health, Regain Strength, Live longer.* New York, NY: McGraw-Hill. 2007. [Lymphedema can happen from lymph node removal, particularly if the area receives radiation. p. 44]. [Survivors with a history of any type tissue-graft reconstruction need to know which muscles were repositioned, how that affects mobility, the best ways to stretch, how massages can help, and how to compensate. pp. 81-101]. [Muscular anatomy visuals are provided for each type of breast cancer surgery. Some suggestions are based on strength deficits. Book overview].

82. Kairaluoma PM, Bachmann MS, Rosenberg PH, Pere PJ. "Preincisional Paravertebral Block Reduces the Prevalence of Chronic Pain After Breast Surgery." *Anesthesia & Analgesia*. 2006; 103(3): 703-708.

83. Katz SJ, Lantz, PM, Janz NK, et al. "Patient Involvement in Surgery Treatment Decisions for Breast Cancer." *Journal of Clinical Oncology*. 2005; 23(24): 5526-5533.

84. Kaunitz, Andrew M. "Ramifications of Breast-Conserving Surgery for Ductal Carcinoma in Situ: Ten-Year Follow-Up Shows High Rates of Subsequent Invasive Procedures." Published in Journal Watch Women's Health. 4/26/2012. Summarized from: Nekhlyudov L. et al. "Ten-Year Risk of Diagnostic Mammograms and Invasive Breast Procedures after Breast-Conserving Surgery for DCIS." *Journal of the National Cancer Institute (JNCI)*. 4/18/2012. 104:614. http://womens-health.jwatch.org/cgi/content/full/2012/426/6 Accessed 5/20/2012.

85. Kelly, Janis. "US Breast Cancer Rates No Longer Falling." *Medscape Medical News > Oncology*. Posted 3/8/2011. www.medscape.com/viewarticle/738593 Adapted from *Cancer Epidemiology Biomarkers and Prevention*. 2011; 20(5):733-739. Accessed 4/2/2011.

86. Kerlikowske K, Cook AJ, Buist DS, et al. "Breast Cancer Risk by Breast Density, Menopause, and Postmenopausal Hormone Therapy Use." *Journal of Clinical Oncology*. 2010; 28(24): 3830-3837.

87. Khaleeli AA, Griffith DG, Edwards RH. "The Clinical Presentation of Hypothyroid Myopathy and its Relationship to Abnormalities in Structure and Function of Skeletal Muscles." *Clinical Endocrinology*. 1983; 19(3): 365-376.

88. Khan, SA. "Contralateral Prophylactic Mastectomy: What Do We Know and What Do Our Patients Know." *Journal of Clinical Oncology. Editorial*. 2011; 29(16): 2132-2135. Published ahead of print www.jco.org 4/4/2011. http://jco. ascopubs.org/content/29/16/2132.full Accessed 8/9/2011.

89. Kharrazian, Datis. *Why Do I Still Have Thyroid Symptoms? When My Lab Tests Are Normal*. Garden City, New York: Morgan James Publishing, LLC. 2010. [Hypothyroidism might worsen hot flashes; the thyroid gland plays a role in temperature regulation. p. 16].

90. King TA, Sakr R, Patil S, Gurevich I, et al. "Clinical Management Factors Contribute to the Decision for Contralateral Prophylactic Mastectomy." *Journal of Clinical Oncology*. 2011; 29(16): 2158-2164.

91. Kirkpatrick C, Buck H, Ellis S. "Assessment of Adrenal Suppression from Two New Dry Powder Inhaler Formulations of Budesonide Delivered by Clickhaler® Compared with the Pulmicort® Turbuhaler. ®" Posted by *PubMed.gov: US National Library of Medicine National Institute of Health*. PMID: 12737682. http://www.ncbi.nlm.nih.gov/pubmed/12737682 Abstract from *Journal of Aerosol Medicine*. 2003; 16(1): 31-36. Accessed 1/26/2012.

92. Klein I, Ojamaa K, Epstein FH, editor. "Thyroid Hormone and the Cardiovascular System." *New England Journal of Medicine*. 2001; 344(7): 501-509.

93. Kohlstadt, Ingrid, editor. *Food and Nutrients in Disease Management*. Boca Raton, FL: Taylor & Francis Group LLC. 2009. [The text educates medical students about the role nutrition and supplementation can play in medicine. Book overview]. [Symptoms of fibromyalgia and chronic fatigue might benefit from adrenal nutrition and supplementation. p. 559]. [A magnesium deficiency might be present if muscle cramps and constipation accompany asthma. p. 139].

94. *Komen, Susan, Foundation*. http:ww5.komen.org/ ["Risk Factors." http:// ww5.komen.org/breastcancer/researchtabletopics.html#riskfactors Accessed 1/8/2013]. [New Year's Resolutions: Get Active and Lower Your Breast Cancer Risk (December 2010). http://ww5.komen.org/Content.aspx?id=6442452904 Accessed 1/28/2013].

95. Kuijpens JL, Nyklíček I, Louwman MW, Weetman TA, et al. "Hypothyroidism Might Be Related to Breast Cancer in Post-Menopausal Women." *Thyroid.* 2005; 15(11): 1253-1259.

96. Landry, Ann. "Study Highlights Communication 'Breakdowns' in Cancer Care. *Cancer Network: Home of the Journal Oncology.* Reported online ahead of print 4/16/2012. Summarized from a Project of the NCI's Cancer Research Network's Cancer Communication Research Center (CRN CCRC). http://www.cancernetwork.com/nurses/content/article/10165/2066521 Accessed 5/8/2012.

97. Laronga, Christine. "The Changing Face of Mastectomy: Nipple Sparing." *Factors News: Fighting Against Cancer Together.* Spring/Summer 2010. p5.

98. Le GM, O'Malley CD, Glaser SL, et al. "Breast Implants Following Mastectomy in Women with Early-Stage Breast Cancer: Prevalence and Impact on Survival." *Breast Cancer Research.* 2005; 7(2): R184-R193. Posted by *PubMed.gov: US National Library of Medicine National Institute of Health.* DOI: 10.1186/bcr974. http://www.ncbi.nlm.nih.gov/pmc/articles/PMC1064128 PMCID:1064128. Accessed 6/27/2010.

99. Lehman CD, Gatsonis C, Kuhl CK, et al. "MRI Evaluation of the Contralateral Breast in Women with Recently Diagnosed Breast Cancer." *New England Journal of Medicine.* 2007; 356(13): 1295-1303.

100. Leidenius M, Leivonen M, Vironen J, Von Smitten K. "The Consequences of Long-Time Arm Morbidity in Node-Negative Breast Cancer Patients with Sentinel Lymph Node Biopsy or Axillary Clearance." *Journal of Surgical Oncology.* 2005; 92(1): 23-31.

101. Lekakis J, Papamichael C, Alevizaki M, et al. "Flow-Mediated, Endothelium-Dependent Vasodilation is Impaired in Subjects with Hypothyroidism, Borderline Hypothyroidism, and High-Normal Serum Thyrotropin (TSH) Values." *Thyroid.* 1997; 7(3): 411-414.

102. Lewit K, Olsanska S. "Clinical Importance of Active Scars: Abnormal Scars as a Cause of Myofascial Pain." *Journal of Manipulative and Physiological Therapeutics.* 2004; 27(6): 399-402.

103. Loftus L, Laronga C. "Evaluating Patients with Chronic Pain After Breast Cancer Surgery: The Search for Relief." *JAMA.* 2009; 302(18): 2034-2035.

104. Love, Susan M. *Dr. Susan Love's Breast Book.* 4th edition. Cambridge, MA: Da Capo Press. 2005. [Dense tissue is a strong breast cancer risk factor. p. 153]. [Stage I breast cancer has less than a 5% recurrence rate over a five-year period. p. 248]. [Cancer on the opposite breast occurs, on average, to 15% of women. p. 449]. [Lymphedema is a long-term concern, even for women who lose less lymph nodes. p. 455].

105. Luboshitzky R, Herer P, Lavie L. "Cardiovascular Risk Factors in Middle Aged Women with Subclinical Hypothyroidism." *Neuroendocrinology Letters.* www.nel.edu. Aug. 2004; 25(4): 262-266. http://www.nel.edu/pdf_/25_4/NEL250404A03_Luboshitzky_.pdf. Accessed 1/26/2012.

106. Lucas, Geralyn. *Why I Wore Lipstick to My Mastectomy.* New York, NY: St. Martin's Press. 2004. [Ms. Lucas' husband, (also a physician), had difficulties coping with the medical aspects of her breast cancer diagnosis. For a time she had to accept his withdrawal and attend appointments without him. pp. 114-124].

107. Manuel F, Hirschberg G. "Physical Therapy for Post Breast Surgery Pain Syndrome."*CancerLynx: We Prowl the Net.* Reprinted by *Cancerlynx,* with permission from *Cancer Supportive Care.* Posted 5/13/2002. http://www. cancerlynx.com/paintherapy.html Accessed 4/20/2011.

108. Martin, Richard. *St. Petersburg Times:tbt.* "A Mastectomy that is Kinder to the Breast." In Print: Aug. 4th 2009.

109. McCarthy CM, Klassen AF, Cano SJ, et al. "Patient Satisfaction with Post Mastectomy Breast Reconstruction: A Comparison of Saline and Silicone Implants." *Cancer.* 2010; 116(24): 5584-5591.

110. McDonnell SK, Schaid DJ, Myers JL, et al. "Efficacy of Contralateral Prophylactic Mastectomy in Women with a Personal and Family History of Breast Cancer." *Journal of Clinical Oncology.* 2001; 19(19): 3938-3943.

111. Meletis CD, Centrone WA. "Adrenal Fatigue: Enhancing Quality of Life for Patients with a Functional Disorder." *Alternative and Complementary Therapies.* 2002; 8(5): 267-272.

112. Miller, Kenneth D, editor. *Choices in Breast Cancer Treatment: Medical Specialists and Cancer Survivors Tell What You Need to Know.* USA: The Johns Hopkins University Press. 2008. [Most women diagnosed with breast cancer do not have a genetic predisposition, a first-degree relative with breast cancer, or a second-degree relative with the disease. p. 65].

113. Mistry N, Wass J, Turner MR. "When to Consider Thyroid Dysfunction in the Neurology Clinic." *Practical Neurology.* 2009; 9(3):145-156.

114. Monzani F, Caraccio N, Del Guerra P, Casolaro A, Ferrannini E. "Neuromuscular Symptoms and Dysfunction in Subclinical Hypothyroid Patients: Beneficial Effect of L-T4 Replacement Therapy." *Clinical Endocrinology.* 1999; 51(2): 237-242.

115. Moyer Christine. "Has Participatory Medicine's Time Arrived? Professional Issues." *American Medical News.* From AAFP 2010 Scientific Assembly. Published 11/15/2010. pp. 19-20.

116. Mukherjee, Siddhartha. *The Emperor Of All Maladies: A Biography of Cancer.* New York, N.Y: Scribner. 2010. [The breast cancer treatment pendulum has swung from radical surgical, chemical, and radiation approaches, to the minimalist ones that are now the norm. Book overview]. [Close-mindedness kept a survivor from spreading the word about a support group as recently as the early 1950s, when *The New York Times* refused to print the words *breast cancer.* pp. 26-27].

117. Mulcahy, Nick. "NCCN Breast Cancer Guidelines Have 'Major' Changes." *Medscape Medical News: Conference News.* Not sanctioned by, nor a part of, the National Comprehensive Cancer Network. Summarized from the National Comprehensive Cancer Network (NCCN) 17th Annual Conference. Presented 3/16/2012, Hollywood, FL. Posted 3/23/2012. http://www.medscape.com/viewarticle/760802 Accessed 5/14/2012.

118. Mulcahy, Nick. "25-Year Results in Early Breast Cancer Surgery." *Medscape Medical News > Oncology.* http://www.medscape.com/viewarticle/734089 Posted 12/11/2010. Primary source: 33rd Annual San Antonio Breast Cancer Symposium (SABCS): Abstracts P4-10-01 and P4-10-02. Presented 12/11/2010. Accessed 3/23/2011.

119. Murphy, Barbara A. "Do Psychosocial Interventions Reduce Pain in Cancer Patients? A Meta-Analysis Demonstrates Meaningful Effects on Pain Severity and Pain Interference." *Journal Watch Oncology and Hematology.* 2/28/2012. http://oncology-hematology.jwatch.org/cgi/content/full/2012/228/3 Accessed 5/20/2012.

120. Napoli R, Guardasole V, Zarra E, D'Anna C, et al. "Impaired Endothelial—and Non-Endothelial-Mediated Vasodilation in Patients with Acute or Chronic Hypothyroidism." *Clinical Endocrinology.* 2010; 72(1): 107-111.

121. *National Cancer Institute: at the National Institute of Health.* ["Mammograms: False Negative Results" http://www.cancer.gov/cancertopics/factsheet/detection/mammograms Reviewed 9/22/2010. Accessed 5/5/2012]. ["Preventive Double Mastectomies Increasing Despite Some Concerns." http://www.cancer.gov/cancertopics/prevention/breast/preventive-mastectomies1107 Posted 11/01/2007. Accessed 5/19/2011].

122. *National Comprehensive Care Network*: "Updated NCCN Guidelines for Breast Cancer Discourages Prophylactic Mastectomies in Women Other Than Those at High Risk." http://www.nccn.org/about/news/newsinfo.asp?NewsID=226 Posted 10/28/2009. Accessed 5/21/2012.

123. *National Lymphedema Network.* Lymph Question Corner "Risk Reduction Practices." http://www.lymphnet.org/ Posted Apr.-Jun. 2009. Accessed 6/27/2010.

124. Nekhlyudov L, Habel LA, Achacoso N, et al. "Ten-Year risk of Diagnostic Mammograms and Invasive Breast Procedures after Breast-Conserving Surgery for DCIS." *Journal of the National Cancer Institute (JNCI).* 2012; 104(8): 614-621. DOI: 10.1093/jnci/djs167. First published online 4/5/2012. http://jnci.oxfordjournals.org/content/104/8/614 Accessed 5/13/2012.

125. Newman LA. "Nipple-Sparing Mastectomy with Breast Reconstruction." *Medscape Oncology.* Posted 6/25/2010. www.medscape.org/viewarticle/723967 Accessed 1/16/2012.

126. Niederberger E, Kühlein H, Geisslinger G. "Update on the Pathobiology of Neuropathic Pain." *Medscape News.* Posted 1/22/2009. Adapted from *Expert Review of Proteomics.* 2008; 5(6): 799-818. http://www.medscape.com/view-article/586220 Accessed 4/8/2011.

127. Northrup, Christiane. *The Wisdom of Menopause: Creating Physical and Emotional Health During the Change.* New York: Bantam Dell. 2006. [With the exclusion of women with a *new* breast cancer diagnosis, we should perform caring massages to get in touch with ourselves, not militant, fearful breast exams. pp. 459-460]. [A quarter of women develop hypothyroidism during or close to perimenopause, a problem that can be worsened by estrogen therapy. p. 119]. ["There are dozens of medical studies on breast cancer alone showing that feelings of powerlessness in important relationships and an inability to express the full range of emotions raise the risk of developing breast cancer and lower survival rates from it." p. 58].

128. Ørstavik K, Norheim I, Jørum E. "Pain and Small-Fiber Neuropathy in Patients with Hypothyroidism." *Neurology.* 2006; 67(5): 786-791.

129. *Oxford University Press (OUP).* "Spin and Bias in Published Studies of Breast Cancer Trials." *ScienceDaily.* 1/10/2013. http://www.sciencedaily.com/releases/2013/01/130109215234.htm Summarized from "Bias in Reporting of Endpoints of Efficacy and Toxicity in Randomized Clinical Trials for Women with Breast Cancer." *Annals of Oncology,* 2013 DOI: 10.1093/annonc/mds636. Accessed 2/1/2013.

130. Oz, Mehmet. *Healing from the Heart: A Leading Heart Surgeon Explores the Power of Complementary Medicine.* New York: Penguin Books. 1998. [While in China, Dr. Oz was shown how Chinese medicine and Western medicine can work side by side. The clinic triaged patients, then sent them to be treated by one of those two medical models. Neither approach was seen as better, or even mutually exclusive, just different for different diseases. He was told that Western medicine is better for acute problems, and that Chinese medicine might work better for chronic ones. p. 160]. [Complementary therapies, such as meditation, massages, visualizations, and acupuncture, can reduce pain, lower anxiety, and improve outcomes in a clinical setting, particularly in a surgical setting. Book overview].

131. Park CC, Rembert J, Chew K, et al. "High Mammographic Density is Independent Predictor of Local but not Distant Recurrence after Lumpectomy and Radiotherapy for Invasive Breast Cancer." *International Journal of Radiation Oncology* Biology* Physics.* Jan. 2009; 73(1): 75-79. Posted by *PubMed.gov: US National Library of Medicine National Institute of Health.* PMID: 18692323. http://www.ncbi.nlm.nih.gov/pubmed/18692323 Accessed 1/28/2012.

132. Peralta EA, Ellenhorn JD, Wagman LD, Dagis A, Andersen JS, Chu DZ. "Contralateral Prophylactic Mastectomy Improves the Outcome of Selected Patients Undergoing Mastectomy for Breast Cancer." *The American Journal of Surgery.* 2000; Volume 180(6): 439-445.

133. Poleshuck EL, Katz J, Andrus CH, Hogan LA Jung BF, et al. "Risk factors for Chronic Pain Following Breast Cancer Surgery: A Prospective Study." *The Journal of Pain.* 2006; 7(9): 626-634.

134. Rakha EA, Lee AH, Evans AJ, Menon S, et al "Tubular Carcinoma of the Breast: Further Evidence to Support Its Excellent Prognosis." *Journal of Clinical Oncology: Official Journal of the American Society of Clinical Oncology (JCO).* 2010; 28(1): 99-104. Posted by *PubMed.gov: US National Library of Medicine National Institute of Health.* PMID: 19917872. http://www.ncbi.nlm.nih.gov/pubmed/19917872 Accessed 5/14/2012.

135. Raymond, Joan. "Effects of Sexual Abuse Last for Decades, Study Finds: Levels of So-Called Stress Hormone are Altered for Years, Sometimes Causing Physical and Mental Problems, Researchers Find." *More health news on msnbc.com.* Updated 6/30/2011. http://www.msnbc.msn.com/id/43594639/ns/health-health_care/ Accessed 7/1/2011.

136. Roizen Michael F, Oz Mehmet C, with The Joint Commission: The Patient's Safety Champion. *You The Smart Patient: An Insider's Handbook for Getting the Best Treatment.* New York, NY: Free Press. 2006. [Doctors cannot heal us on the spot. We should ask informed questions and become informed about all of our treatments. Information on various types of insurance plans, complementary practitioners' licensures, self-advocacy resources and related websites are included. Book overview]. [One of the most regulated complementary therapies (CAM) in the USA is acupuncture. p. 298].

137. Rolnick SJ, Altschuler A, Nekhlyudov L, et al. "What Women Wish They Knew Before Prophylactic Mastectomy." *Cancer Nursing.* 2007; 30(4): 285-291.

138. Rothfeld Glenn S, Romaine Deborah S. *Thyroid Balance: Traditional and Alternative Methods for Treating Thyroid Disorders.* Avon, MA: Adams Media. 2003. [Hypothyroidism symptoms can resemble some menopause symptoms. p. 179]. [One half of patients with hypothyroidism might develop adrenal insufficiencies. p. 92]. [Radiation in proximity to the thyroid gland, and poor nutrition due to chemotherapy, might affect thyroid function directly or indirectly; patients undergoing cancer treatments should have thyroid screenings twice a year. p. 247]. ["Once adrenal fatigue seems under control, it's sometimes necessary to adjust the thyroid hormone supplement." p. 102].

139. Rowan, K. "Breast Cancer Risk Linked to Breast Density.*" My Health News Daily, MSNBC.* Updated 10/7/2010. http://www.msnbc.msn.com/id/39556386/ns/health-cancer Accessed 3/19/2011.

140. Schmitz KH, Ahmed RL, Troxel AB, Cheville A, Lewis-Grant L, Smith R, et al. "Weight Lifting for Women at Risk for Breast Cancer-Related Lymphedema: A Randomized Trial." *JAMA.* 2010; 304(24): 2699-2705.

141. Schwenk, Thomas, L. "Ultrasound Plus Mammography for Breast Cancer Screening." Adapted from *Journal Watch (General)* 2008; 7(5) © 2008. www.medscape.com/viewarticle/575416 Posted 07/21/2008. Accessed 4/2/2011.

142. Selim S, Shapiro R, Hwang SE, et al. "Post Breast Therapy Pain Syndrome (PBTPS)." *Cancer Supportive Care Programs*. http://www.cancersupportivecare.com/neuropathicpain.php Updated 10/31/2007. Accessed 3/24/2011.

143. Shames Richard L, Shames Karilee H. *Thyroid Power: 10 Steps to Total Health.* New York, NY: Harper Collins. 2005. [Fatigue and mental clarity difficulties can be symptoms of hypothyroidism. p. 56]. [Adrenal imbalances happen *gradually*—like Hans Selye's general adaptation syndrome. Adrenal treatment should be based on the stage the patient is experiencing. pp. 135-138].

144. Shockney, Lillie. *Navigating Breast Cancer; A Guide for the Newly Diagnosed.* Sudbury MA: Jones and Bartlet Publishers, LLC. 2007.

145. Shomon Mary J. *The Menopause Thyroid Solution: Overcoming Menopause by Solving Your Hidden Thyroid Problems.* New York, NY: Harper Collins. 2009. [Symptoms from hypothyroidism, perimenopause, and from menopause are alike and develop during similar life stages, making an adequate diagnosis difficult. Even women who are not overweight might suffer from hypothyroidism. pp. 6-9]. [Hypothyroidism can cause hypotension and hypertension. p. 46]. [In 2003, the American Association of Clinical Endocrinologists recommended doctors aim for TSH levels of 0.3 to 3.0. p. 117]. [Thyroid levels should be monitored if steroids, some antidepressants, or select anticonvulsants are prescribed. They might be metabolized differently in individuals with hypothyroidism, increasing hypothyroid symptoms or medication side effects. pp. 121-123]. [Surgical or medical menopause, steroid use and stress, can interfere with thyroid function. pp. 122 & 134].

146. Siegel, Bernie S. *Love, Medicine & Miracles: Lessons Learned About Self-Healing from a Surgeon's Experience with Exceptional Patients.* New York: Harper Collins. 1986. [To maximize emotional and physical healing, cancer patients must eventually ask "Why did I need the illness?" pp. 108-112]. ["Exceptional patients do indeed want to be educated and want to be made "doctors" of their own cases." "One of the most important roles that they demand of their physicians is that of a teacher." p. 27].

147. Siegel, Bernie S. *Peace Love & Healing; Body Mind Communication and the Path to Self-Healing: An Exploration.* New York: Harper Collins. 1989. ["Gifts" are available to patients who do the emotional and the spiritual work of cancer. p. 190]. [Negative influences from early years, including every type of abuse, sense of loneliness, or feelings of not being loved adequately, tend to create over-pleasing personalities and predispositions to illnesses such as cancer later in life. Cancer patients should express their negative emotions. "When you put your feelings outside, you may heal inside. And you will certainly heal your life, if not your disease." pp. 159-161. Quote p. 158].

148. Silver, Mark. *Breast Cancer Husband: How to Help Your Wife (and Yourself) through Diagnosis, Treatment, and Beyond.* U.S.A: Holtzbrinck Publishers. 2004. [Breast cancer partners function as supporters, even if they do not agree with medical decisions. Since needs vary, couples should determine how the well spouse can be of assistance. pp. 98-104].

149. Simpson, Kathy R. *Overcoming Adrenal fatigue.* Oakland, CA: New Harbinger Publications. 2009. [If thyroid medication is taken during an adrenal insufficiency symptoms can worsen. p. 92]. [Cortisol is necessary for thyroid hormone conversion and utilization. p. 94]. [Hydrocortisone is at least five times less powerful than Prednisone. p. 77]. [Over exercising through adrenal insufficiency further taxes the endocrine system. p. 112]. [Licorice root can help stabilize cortisol levels, but it might raise blood pressure. p. 74]. [Asthma and allergies can be worsened by adrenal insufficiencies. p. 35].

150. Stabouli S, Papakatsika S, Kotsis V. "Hypothyroidism and Hypertension." *Medscape.com.* Posted 12/26/2010. Summarized from *Expert Review of Cardiovascular Therapy.*" 2010; 8(11): 1559-1565. http://www.medscape.com/viewarticle/733788 Accessed 4/24/2011.

151. Steligo, Kathy. *The Breast Reconstruction Guide Book: Issues and Answers from Research to Recovery.* San Carlos, CA: Carlo Press. 2003. [NSM "leaves potentially harmful cells behind." p. 23]. [If contoured implants rotate, surgery is necessary to reposition them. p. 83].

152. Stevens WG, Pacella SJ, Gear AJ, et al. "Clinical Experience with a Fourth-Generation Textured Silicone Gel Breast Implant: a Review of 1012 Mentor Memory Gel Breast Implants." *Aesthetic Surgery Journal: The American Society for Aesthetic Plastic Surgery.* 2008; 28(6): 642-647.

153. Stubblefield MD, Custodio CM. "Upper-Extremity Pain Disorders in Breast Cancer." *Archives of Physical Medicine and Rehabilitation.* 2006; 87(3) Supplement 1: S96-S99.

154. Tabár L, Vitak B, Chen TH, et al. "Swedish Two-County Trial: Impact of Mammographic Screening on Breast Cancer Mortality During 3 Decades." *Radiology.* Sept. 2011; 260(3): 658-63. Posted by *PubMed.gov: US National Library of Medicine National Institute of Health.* DOI: 10.1148/radiol.11110469. PMID: 21712474. http://www.ncbi.nlm.nih.gov/pubmed/21712474 Accessed 1/21/2012.

155. Tasmuth T, Von Smitten K, Hieatanen P, et al. "Pain and Other Symptoms after Different Treatment Modalities of Breast Cancer." *Annals of Oncology.* 1995; 6(5): 453-459.

156. Throckmorton AD, Esserman LJ. "When Informed, All Women Do Not Prefer Breast Conservation." *Journal of Clinical Oncology: Editorial.* 2009; 27(4): 484-486.

157. Tosovic A, Bondeson AG, Bondeson L, Ericcson UB, et al. "Prospectively Measured Triiodothyronine Levels Are Positively Associated with Breast Cancer Risk in Postmenopausal Women." *Breast Cancer Research: Open Access.* 2010; 12(3): R33.DOI:10.1186/bcr2587. http://breast-cancer-research.com/content/12/3/R33 Accessed 5/17/2012.

158. Tuttle TM, Habermann EB, Grund EH, Morris TJ, Virnig BA. "Increasing Use of Contralateral Prophylactic Mastectomy for Breast Cancer Patients: A Trend Toward More Aggressive Surgical Treatment." *Journal of Clinical Oncology*. 2007; 25(33): 5203-5209.

159. Tuttle, TM. "Counseling Breast Cancer Patients on Contralateral Prophylactic Mastectomy: The Physician's Role." *Oncology (Willston Park)*. 2008; 22(5): 545-8. Posted by *PubMed.gov: US National Library of Medicine National Institute of Health*. PMID: 18533403. http://www.ncbi.nlm.nih.gov/pubmed?term=18533403 Accessed 1/11/2012.

160. Ueda S, Tamaki Y, Yano K, Okishiro N, Yanagisawa T, et al. "Cosmetic Outcome and Patient Satisfaction after Skin-Sparing Mastectomy for Breast Cancer with Immediate Reconstruction of the Breast." *Surgery*. 2008; 143(3): 414-25. Posted by *PubMed.gov: US National Library of Medicine National Institute of Health*. 12/21/2007. PMID: 18291263. http://www.ncbi.nlm.nih.gov/pubmed/18291263 Accessed 5/10/2012.

161. *U.S. Department of Health and Human Services: National Endocrine and Metabolic Diseases Information Service. A Service of the National Institute of Diabetes and Digestive and Kidney Diseases (NIDDK), National Institutes of Health (NIH)*. "Adrenal Insufficiency and Addison's Disease." http://endocrine.niddk.nih.gov/pubs/addison/addison.aspx Publication No. 09-3054. May 2009. Accessed 10/15/2010.

162. *University of California Davis Health System*. "Second Lumpectomy For Breast Cancer Reduces Survival Rates. Summarized from "The Survival Impact of the Choice of Surgical Procedure after Ipsilateral Breast Cancer. "*The American Journal of Surgery*. 2008; 196(4) 495-499. http://www.ucdmc.ucdavis.edu/welcome/features/20081210_2ndLumpectomy/index.html Accessed 5/30/2011.

163. *Value-Based Cancer Care: Integrating Providers, Payers, and the Entire Oncology Team*. "Contralateral Prophylactic Mastectomies Improves Survival, is Cost Effective in Some." Primary source: 2010 ASCO Breast Cancer Symposium. Report by investigators of the Mayo Clinic, Rochester, MN. http://valuebasedcancer.com/article/contralateral-prophylactic-mastectomy-improves-survival-is-cost-effective-for-some Accessed 3/21/2011.

164. Van Duijnhoven FJ, Peeters PH, Warren RM, et al. "Postmenopausal Hormone Therapy and Changes in Mammographic Density." *Journal of Clinical Oncology*. 2007; 25(11): 1323-1328.

165. Vidt, DG. "Thyroid Dysfunction and Hypertension: What's the Connection?" *Cleveland Clinic Foundation*. Posted 1/1/2004. http://consultantlive.com/hypertension/content/article/10162/45704 Accessed 5/23/2010.

166. Walker AE, Gelfand A, Katon WJ, et al. "Adult Health Status of Women with Histories of Childhood Abuse and Neglect." *The American Journal of Medicine*. 1999; 107(4): 332-339.

167. Waknine, Yael. "Mammography Benefits Outweigh Risk in Some 40- to 49-Year-Olds."*MedScape Nurses News*. Posted 5/1/2012. Summarized from: Van Ravesteyn N, Miglioretti DL, et al. "Tipping the Balance of Benefits and Harms to Favor Screening Mammography Starting at Age 40 Years: A Comparative Modeling Study of Risk."*Annals of Internal Medicine*. 2012; 156(9): 609-617, 635-648 & 662-663. http://www.medscape.com/view-article/763017 Accessed 5/10/2012.

168. Wang SH, Chu H, Shamliyan T, Jalal H, et al. "Network Meta-analysis of Margin Threshold for Women with Ductal Carcinoma In Situ." *Journal of the National Cancer Institute (JNCI). Oxford Journals: Medicine*. 2012; 104(7):507-516. First published on line 3/22/2012. http://jnci.oxfordjournals.org/content/104/7/507 Accessed 5/15/2012.

169. Wascher, RA, Rosenbaum EH, et al. Post Breast Therapy Pain Syndrome Handout. Posted 2/28/2005. http://www.cancerlynx.com/pbtpshandout.html Accessed 1/26/2011.

170. Weil, Andrew. *You Can't Afford To Get Sick: Your Guide to Optimum Health and Health Care*. New York, NY: Penguin Group. 2009. [A more integrative approach to medicine would reduce health care costs, might encourage research to understand diseases instead of focusing on masking symptoms, could reduce drug toxicities, and would encourage patients to become more involved in finding solutions. The idea that healing takes place overnight prompts unnecessary procedures, medicines and expense. Our present fee-based system is benefitting neither patients nor physicians, but change is taking place. A third of medical schools are "members of the Consortium of Academic Health Centers for Integrative Medicine (www.imconsortium.org)." Book overview. Quote p. 113].

171. Weiss Marisa, Weiss Ellen. *Living Well Beyond Breast Cancer: A Survivors Guide for When Treatment Ends and the Rest of Your Life Begins*. New York: Three River Press. 2010. [Useful self-involvement suggestions, including how to choose health care providers, and detailed information on pharmaceuticals to manage long-term pain are provided. Book overview]. [Cancer on the opposite breast is considered a new cancer, not necessarily a recurrence. A new cancer (or a second primary) can also happen on the already-treated breast, and it too might be excluded from recurrence statistics. p. 447]. [Nerves can be compressed by scar tissue. p. 176].

172. *Western New England College. Engineering Challenges: See the Future Through the Eyes of an Engineer.* "Design a Torso Positioning Device for Pre-Operative Planning of Breast Reconstructive Surgery." 2009; 12(1): 3.

173. Wilson, James, L. *Adrenal Fatigue: The 21st Century Stress Syndrome.* Petaluma, CA: Smart Publications. 2001. [Low cortisol levels can cause weight loss, fatigue, hypoglycemia and low blood pressure. pp. 61-64]. [Adrenal insufficiency might not be noticed until a major stressor, such as surgery. p. 230]. [Most traditional practitioners don't recognize adrenal insufficiencies until they are more advanced, or believe in integrative approaches to test or treat the condition. pp. 53-54]. [Adding moderate amounts of vitamin C, homeopathic remedies, vitamin E, and B vitamins, particularly B6, might help adrenal insufficiencies. pp. 193-202]. [Eating frequent meals (starting with breakfast), and adding fresh fruits, vegetables, protein and complex carbohydrates, can also go a long way. Avoiding caffeine, alcohol, refined sugars, fried foods, might also make a difference. pp. 133-173].

174. Yi M, Meric-Bernstram F, Middleton LP, Arun BK, Bedrosian I, et al. "Predictors of Contralateral Breast Cancer in Patients with Unilateral Breast Cancer Undergoing Contralateral Mastectomy." *Cancer.* 2009; 115(5): 962-971.

175. Zimmerman, Ron. "Double Whammy: Unemployment After Breast Cancer Diagnosis." *Medscape Medical News WebMD.* Posted 12/9/2011. Primary source: 34th San Antonio Breast Cancer Symposium (SABCS); Abstract #PD06-09. Presented 12/9/2011. http://www.medscape.com/viewarticle/755196 Accessed 5/20/2012.

176. Ziv E, Tice J, Smith-Bindman R, et al. "Mammographic Density and Estrogen Receptor Status of Breast Cancer." *Cancer Epidemiology, Biomarkers & Prevention.* 2004; 13(12): 2090-2095

Index

www.ingramcontent.com/pod-product-compliance
Lightning Source LLC
Chambersburg PA
CBHW022104280326
41933CB00007B/252